THE
PHILOSOPHY &
PRACTICE OF YOGA

Roy Eugene Davis is founder-director of Center for Spiritual Awareness, a New Era truth movement with an international outreach. He began his spiritual training with Paramahansa Yogananda in 1950. Mr. Davis is the editor-publisher of *Truth Journal* magazine, author of many inspirational books and a world-traveled teacher of meditation methods and how-to-live principles.

ROY EUGENE DAVIS
COLLECTED WRITINGS
Volume Two

THE
PHILOSOPHY &
PRACTICE OF YOGA

CSA PRESS, *Publishers*
Lakemont, Georgia 30552

*Copyright © 1976
by Roy Eugene Davis*

THIS EDITION 1983

This title is Volume Two of the Collected Writings Series. Contact the Publisher for a complete list of other available titles by the author: CSA Press, Post Office Box 7, Lakemont, Georgia 30552. CSA Press is the literature department of Center for Spiritual Awareness.

MANUFACTURED IN THE UNITED STATES OF AMERICA

I salute the supreme teacher, the Truth, whose nature is bliss, who is the giver of the highest happiness, who is pure wisdom, who is beyond all qualities and infinite like the sky, who is beyond words, who is one and eternal, pure and still, who is beyond all change and phenomena and who is the silent witness to all our thoughts and emotions—I salute Truth, the supreme teacher.

—Ancient Vedic Hymn

CONTENTS

Foreword	9
Yoga and Yogic Systems	13
The Nature of the World and Stages of Self-Realization	29
Purification of the Body	46
Asanas for Health and Mastery	50
Pranayamas for Regulating Vital Forces	64
Mudras: Awakening Kundalini and Acquiring Conscious Control Over the Involuntary Nervous System	68
Yogic Initiation and Meditation Techniques	81
Suggested Routines of Practice	89
The Message of the Siddhas	95
Masters of Yoga	101
Glossary	183

FOREWORD

There are many useful and popular books on yoga which have been widely distributed, and which serve well. This offering is meant as a guide to the sincere and dedicated seeker on the path, whose yearning for liberation of consciousness is intense. In short, this book is for one who wants to be an embodiment of yoga.

Because of the intimate presentation of this material, the reader will find *The Philosophy and Practice of Yoga* to be a personal guide on the path. Yoga is not for the over-anxious, and it most assuredly is not for that person who is lazy. Yoga is for that special type of person who is willing to give his all to the disciplines leading to self-transformation and enlightenment.

While I have purposely avoided many of the extreme claims found in some original texts, I have presented the subject truly and in a concise manner. Some Sanskrit words have been included, both for the purpose of introducing the vital message and because of the *mantra* power they possess and impart. One need not adopt another cultural lifestyle in order to practice yoga, but it is well, I feel, for one to enter fully into the tradition in order to derive highest benefits.

The purpose of yogic disciplines is to cleanse the body, mind and consciousness of everything which prevents the free flow of soul awareness. To cleanse the body, we do certain things to encourage the removal of waste matters; to cleanse the mind, we release and neutralize patterns which do not serve a higher purpose; to refine the brain and nervous system, we let in the light of superconsciousness so that the final work can be accomplished. This is the essence of yoga. Yoga, according to the classic text, the *Bhagavad-Gita,* is for the determined, the courageous, the truly dedicated. It is not for one who engages in the various procedures without conscious intent or because of a need for something to do as a change from boring routine. As practitioners of yoga, we are motivated to awaken from the dream of mortality and awaken fully to our divine nature.

I have written of my own spiritual discipline *(sadhana)* practiced under the guidance of my guru, Paramahansa Yogananda, in my spiritual autobiography. A brief account will also be found in the pages of this present book. Yoga is both a philosophy and a procedure which reveals the light of Truth. Hence, it is referred to as *yoga darsana. Darsana* (darshan) means "vision of light" or "the light that is revealed." It also refers to the philosophy of life that reveals the highest truth. The great seers consider *darsana* as more than speculative philosophical examination. Rather, one is to study, contemplate and realize the essence of truth which inspired a philosophical conclusion. The correct approach, then, is to examine the teaching and test the principles in order to experience insight and realization.

Many of the readers of this treatise will be initiates of Kriya Yoga or of another yogic tradition. For them this material will be of great value. Here is the complete system of yoga as taught by the *siddhas,* the masters who have realized perfection. I would suggest, as a practical approach, a complete reading of the book, then a systematic study, followed by practice of the procedures. Yoga can only be truly known by one who engages in the process.

It is true that one who becomes a successful yogi attains *siddhis,* the powers of perfection. These are not to be used without discrimination, but only as the intelligence of God within directs.

The second part of the book is devoted to a number of short biographical accounts of a few known *siddha* masters. It is my hope that this addition will prove to be of inspirational and motivational importance to the reader.

A teaching tradition is a matter of emphasis, but the basic philosophy and program of discipline is common to all on the yoga path. Gurus teach according to inner guidance, to meet practical needs of disciples and to meet them at their level of need, based on an understanding of the disciple's psychological temperament and aptitude.

I acknowledge, with appreciation, the support and cooperation of friends and disciples who have been helpful in the preparation of the manuscript. My thanks, too, go to Baba Haridas, Mr. K.K. Sah (Naini Tal, Himalayas) and Subhash Mahajan for useful data concerning some of the *siddhas* whose work is explained in the latter pages. Ron Lindahn took the photographs of me doing *yogasanas* and other procedures. Everyone whose life I have been privileged to touch has played a role in this finished work.

Roy Eugene Davis

Lakemont, Georgia
June 24, 1983

Chapter One
YOGA AND YOGIC SYSTEMS

Wherever there are persons who practice an intentional discipline leading to Self-Mastery and the enlightenment experience, there Yoga is practiced. Yogic teachings predate recorded history, but it is in India that the first records were made concerning man's experiments to control the mind, become Self-actualized and awaken to the realization of the Truth concerning the nature of Consciousness.

It is taught that knowledge of a thing is inherent in the thing and that knowledge of a scientific process is inherent in the process itself. When the worlds were formed, the knowledge of the worlds emerged from the same Source. Since we came from the Source into outer involvement with nature, we carry within us the knowledge of the process. Yoga practice is designed to create a situation whereby one will be able to recall consciously the truth of his own being and to comprehend the workings of the universe. In this tradition, we teach that truth is revealed from within, for if truth were not already innate, we would not be able to grasp or accept it when confronted by it.

Yoga derives from *yuj*: "to join, to bind, to yoke." It offers one the opportunity of regulating inner processes, restraining urges, focusing attention and awakening to conscious awareness of the true nature. No matter how useful the practice might be, one who practices *Yogasanas* a few times a week, for the health benefits only, is not a yogi. One who "does Yoga" now and then is not a yogi. A yogi is a person who is totally involved in the process and whose goal is Liberation of Consciousness. All others are adapting some of the exercises to their personal requirements but cannot be considered yogis. A male is a yogi or yogin; a female is a yogini. Both male and female are equally endowed with the potential for success in Yoga, and the difference in designation has to do with language usage only.

Lord Shiva, the guiding intelligence of the Holy Spirit aspect of the Godhead, is considered by Indian yogis to be the first teacher of this sacred science. *Brahma* is the aspect of the Godhead which is initial cause and is expansive; *Vishnu* is the aspect of the Godhead which preserves order and maintains balance; *Shiva* is the aspect of the Godhead which flows into expression as the universe and, after a time, dissolves the universe. The *Shiva* aspect also is concerned with removing the clouds of *maya* from the mind and the consciousness of devotees of God. *Brahma, Vishnu* and *Shiva* coincide with the Christian concept of the Trinity, the triple characteristics of the Godhead: God the Father, God the Son (Christ Consciousness), God the Holy Spirit. Their functions are identical.

Shiva is called "King of Yogis" and is the patron deity of Yoga. *Shiva* is portrayed as being forever established in yogic meditation. Various symbols adorn the paintings of this sage: the new moon in his hair represents the dawn of Enlightenment; the cobra around his neck represents awakened and mastered *kundalini*; the female figure in his hair represents *shakti*, the feminine creative energy in nature which has become united with *shakta*, the male principle; the water being sent forth by *shakti* represents the vital force being sent out for the transformation of the worlds; the trident represents *sushumna, ida* and *pingala*, the central spinal nerve and the left and right channels beside it, which are worked within Yogic practice. *Shiva* wears *rudraksha* beads, and his outer symbol is the *lingam*, set before him and representing both the mutation of Consciousness from the unmanifest to the manifest and the union of *shiva-shakti*, which makes possible the worlds. His abode is the Himalayas, far removed from the restless activities of unenlightened society. Yet *Shiva*, the Holy Spirit, is easily accessible to those whose preparation and devotion make them fit to receive God's instruction and grace. A *mantra* used when contemplating *Shiva*, the Holy Spirit, is *"Om Namah Shivaya."* We shall discuss *mantras* later in this section.

For one whose *karmic* roots are in India, the close involvement with traditional yogic symbolism will be natural and useful. For one who feels little affinity with this symbolism, I would suggest a sympathetic study and understanding of it, while being true to natural inclinations and to current social mores. One can outwardly conform to any religious form which is meaningful—or to none, according to need and design. Yoga is a discipline, not a religion. We speak of Ultimate Reality and of man's relationship to God, and we recommend an approach to prayer and meditation which is both practical and scientific.

Requirements for the Practice of Yoga

There are at least three prime essentials to be considered by a person who is intent upon success in Yoga practice. First, one must be resolved to commit one's life totally to the discipline, for, as we have said, Yoga is not a part-time practice. Second, one must acquire correct information regarding the philosophy, the systems and the procedures. To be ill-informed or to be superficially informed is a hindrance on the path. Third, one should have a teacher who has attained success in Yoga. There are a few rare souls who have the native aptitude to go it alone, and there are some who are born with Knowledge; most will require personal instruction.

The word *guru* is often loosely translated to mean "teacher." From the roots *gu*—"darkness" and *ru*—"light," a *guru* is one who is able to dispel darkness from the mind and consciousness of the seeker. For awakening of *kundalini* and guidance along the subtle levels during meditation, one will require a *Sat-Guru*, a fully enlightened master of Yoga. In this tradition, it is taught that the *Guru* resides within the seeker's own consciousness as the Guiding Intelligence. A true *guru* will not take advantage of a disciple, nor will he do anything which is not intended for the disciple's liberation. Knowing the way to liberation of the spirit, a *guru* guides the disciple to liberation. One who is not capable of this type of assistance cannot be a true *guru*. The *guru* is truly a spiritual friend who encourages the disciple to do the needed work on the path of Yoga. He also points out self-deception on the part of the disciple or growing lapse in needed disciplines. There is a deeper relationship between *guru* and disciple, when the conditions are ideal. The consciousness and the energy of the *guru* actually enters the disciple to quicken energies and to cleanse mind and consciousness. This is why the disciple must respect and have faith in the *guru*. Without respect and faith, there can be no deep relationship. There must be integrity in the relationship, for a disciple may change teachers but never his *guru*. Should a disciple be left without his *guru's* presence for a time, the telepathic contact can be maintained. If the *guru* is not physically present because of having made his transition, the disciple can be led to an embodied *guru* of the same tradition for personal instruction.

We can and should respect all authentic spiritual traditions, but in Yoga we remain attuned to our own particular line of teachers and *gurus*. Then, the frequency of energy-consciousness to which we have come can result in mental, emotional and spiritual support to us, while we are engaged in our disciplines (*sadhana*) and our practices. One may temporarily forsake the *guru*, but the *guru* never forsakes the disciple. The *guru* is always willing to help and to encourage, but the disciple must be open and receptive.

Hatha Yoga: The Foundation

Not all yogic traditions insist upon the student practicing Hatha Yoga. A *guru* will, of course, teach what he feels is needed for the disciple. But Hatha Yoga is the foundation of all Yoga systems, and one is well-advised to practice the recommended techniques and methods to acquire proficiency, to learn firsthand the effects of such practice and to strengthen the body and the mind for what is to come. In the opening verse of *Hatha Yoga Pradipika*, a classic text, we read: "Reverence to Shiva the Lord of Yoga, who taught (his wife) Parvati Hatha wisdom as the first step to the pinnacle of Raja Yoga." Hatha Yoga, then, is not a separate Yoga: it is the preparation for higher Yogas. *Ha* means "sun" and *tha* means "moon." Thus, Hatha Yoga refers to positive (sun) and to negative (moon) currents in the system. These currents are to be balanced and mastered so that vital force, *prana*, can be regulated, the mind cleared and superconscious states experienced.

The ideal way to practice the Hatha Yoga poses (*asanas*) is to approach the practice session in a calm, meditative mood. Sit quietly for a few moments, then begin the series, slowly, with control and grace, being inwardly aware as the body performs the various poses selected for the practice session. Under no circumstances should there be undue effort, strain or any attempt to compete with others who might be in the class (if one is learning in a group situation). If one takes classes in Hatha Yoga, once the routines have been mastered, the poses can be practiced privately. Since Yoga is an inner process, we do not require the aid or encouragement of others after we have been correctly instructed.

Bhakti Yoga: The Yoga of Love

Without devotion to the ideal, steadiness on the path is unlikely, and, without love and surrender, the ego will hardly be dissolved. Bhakti Yoga is the system in which love and devotion are emphasized. There are Bhakti Yoga traditions which do not teach *asana, pranayama, mudra* or controlled meditation. Love of God, love of God in man, and surrender to God's will is stressed in the Bhakti Yoga approach. One may assume:

"I think I'll give Bhakti Yoga a try!" But, who is trying? In Bhakti Yoga, there is no trying, there is surrender and absorption in the Divine. Some are naturally inclined by temperament to be devotional and to love God and God-as-the-world. Balance is recommended: devotion balanced with reason, love balanced with understanding.

Some bhakti yogins live quietly, with little or no outer evidence of their devotional attitude. Others are more demonstrative, especially while at prayer or worship. Some find that external aids can contribute to a devotional attitude: an altar used during prayer and meditation; pictures of saints to serve as inspiration; chanting or singing; use of *mantra* or even a simple devotional ceremony to aid in creating a mood as preparation for meditation. Whatever a person's approach, if that approach is useful in the long run, it is perfectly in order for him, even though it may not appeal to another.

Singing the names of God aloud can elevate consciousness, clear the mind and even charge the environment with pure energy. For persons who find it difficult to concentrate during meditation and for whom the approach of calm discernment is too subtle, prayer and chanting can be of value.

It is in our day to day life that Bhakti Yoga is truly practiced. Are we loving, compassionate and fair in our dealings with others? All people are endowed with divinity and are deserving of equal respect and caring. To chant God's name in the privacy of the home sanctuary but to mistreat people during other times is not to be a true bhakti yogin. St. Francis is one of the Christian tradition who exemplified the Yoga of love and devotion. Jesus stated the ideal of Bhakti Yoga when he taught, "As you have loved me, love one another." When true love reigns, there can be no barriers; then harmony and fulfillment rule.

When in prayer, any name one uses for God is acceptable. God is what God is; the names we use for God are ours. Simple, direct prayer is the most effective—

just talking with God, then being still. The teaching is that God does not exercise whims in a relationship with man, but by devotion and receptivity we can open ourselves to the Reality of God and attract God's consciousness into our own. Love and devotion also purifies human nature and cleanses the mind and the emotional field. There can be no hate, dislike, jealousy, envy, fear or prejudice in the loving heart. Truly, blessed are the pure in heart, for they can perceive the Reality of God.

Karma Yoga: the Yoga of Selfless Action

Can we ever act selflessly? Yes, we can if our understanding is mature. Who acts? Our Life, which is the Supreme Consciousness, animates mind and body; therefore, the One Life performs all actions. The message of Karma Yoga is this: when we work in harmony with the Power that runs the universe, we are not egotistically motivated, and we no longer maintain compulsive desires relative to the future. With the eradication of compulsive desire, we are able to live in the present, while planning for the future, without being bound to the future. Every reasonable desire carries within itself the motive force for its fulfillment. That is, if an experience is possible to have in this natural world, and we desire it, we are subconsciously pushed toward it or attract it to ourselves.

Yogic philosophy does not say to give up intelligent planning; it says to renounce egotistic desire. We are then able to be open to inner guidance and to flow in the stream of grace. The Intelligence-Power that sustains the universe has a plan and a purpose. When we are in harmony with It we are free, even while involved. One need not leave the world to be free of bondage. One need only see clearly what the world-process is all about and play the role intended in a conscious manner. By doing what we are best suited to do, with understanding, we afford an opportunity for the working out (and neutralizing) of subconscious patterns. Thus, we pay our debt to nature. Our parents provided us with a body. We were cared for and educated by those who took responsibility for us. We have the bounty of nature to enjoy and to utilize wisely. Therefore, it is our duty to assist others as well as nature in the evolutionary process. Not to do this is to shirk our duty, and one who avoids his duty is not fit for the practice of Yoga. This is the teaching, straight and pure.

Even when we find our practices fruitful and our lifestyle in harmony with nature and society, we may find there are deeper instincts and urges yet to be handled and understood. These deep patterns, arising from the unconscious, will eventually have to be released and (or) neutralized; otherwise, we will have no permanent peace. When the conscious level of mind is well-ordered and the subconscious level is cleansed and coordinated with conscious mind intent, there may yet be unconscious patterns to face, in the near or distant future. Only when these patterns on the deep level are released will the soul be free from the possibility of future pain and challenge. One who has become stable in Yoga and is permanently anchored in the realization of God, yet retaining residual *karma* (subconscious impressions-*samsaras*) which will be exhausted in this life cycle, is known as one who is liberated while yet embodied—a free soul (*jivan-mukti*). Such a one is under no compulsion from *karma* to return to this plane of experience. Yet, even while permanently self-realized and established in true knowledge, the body may be affected by the results of residual *karma*, which is working out or being dissipated.

Some, who are not possessed of understanding regarding the inner workings relative to the process of soul liberation, may judge by appearances, when seeing an enlightened person who has a few personal challenges to confront. They might ask: "Why does an enlightened person occasionally become ill, wear glasses or seem to have personality traits which seem inconsistent with the enlightenment experience?" There is an explanation, and we have given it—but it will not satisfy everyone who inquires. A Zen master, in response to such questions, might either try to explain the situation, or he might simply suggest that the questioner mind his own business and get on with his own enlightenment experience.

As we work with a cheerful attitude, doing what we are best suited to do, we know a harmony and an inner peace which those who strive and struggle can never know. We do not feel superior because we have found our right place, however, for this would be pride and evidence of ego.

Deep meditation, especially when *shakti* becomes active, results in deep patterns being flushed to the surface and the experience of cleansing or catharsis. This cleansing can be dramatic, or it can be subtle. Enlightened insight also enables us to see through false concepts which formerly held us in bondage. Then, too, high frequency energies can flow through the nervous system and pervade the entire organism, resulting in purification of the vehicles.

All of the yogic systems are compatible, so that a Yoga of synthesis is the ideal for the mature disciple. With an attitude of surrender, we can open our mind and our heart and ask: "Show me through inner guidance and outer opportunity the way I should go to serve best the cause of world enlightenment. Not my will, O Lord, but your will, be done!"

Jnana Yoga: The Yoga of Knowledge

Those who teach in the tradition of *Jnana Yoga* often state: "Liberation is attained, not by works or ceremony, but by knowledge alone." *Knowledge* in this context is not belief or collected data: it is *comprehension* as a result of discernment and experience. One who truly knows does not affirm, "I believe I know," for this knowledge is a certainty. The Way of Knowledge is for the special few who are prepared for steady examination and clear perception of the nature of Consciousness. In his dissertation on Self-Knowledge (*Atma-Bode*) Shankara begins: "I am composing this treatise on Self-Knowledge to serve the needs of those who have been purified through the practice of spiritual disciplines, who are peaceful in heart, free from (selfish) cravings and desirous of liberation." The *jnana yogin* examines the nature of Supreme Consciousness, God, the soul, and the world-process and, with discernment, clearly sees the truth about it all. His conclusion is the summation of *Vedanta* (the essence of the Vedas): Supreme Consciousness alone is the Reality; any other consideration is the result of faulty perception.

One who chooses this path studies the conclusions of the seers by reading the great scriptures and commentaries, then examining them in the light of his own intelligence and coming to his own realization. In deep meditation, he contemplates the characteristics of Consciousness in manifestation and, by doing so, gains insight and perfect realization.

A great exponent of *Jnana Yoga* in recent times was Ramana Maharshi of southern India. In early years, he underwent spontaneous *kundalini* experience and intense inner purification. Later, as one stable in wisdom, he seldom discussed his early experiences. He acknowledged the usefulness of *shakti* activity, as well as the usefulness of the *guru* for one on the path, but his public emphasis was on examining the true nature of Consciousness by inquiring, "Who am I?" and tracing this back to the Source, Pure Consciousness.

Raja Yoga: The Royal Way

While Yoga was taught and practiced for thousands of years before the advent of Patanjali, it was he who organized the disciplines of mind control and meditative techniques into an orderly treatise known as the *Yoga Sutras*. *Raja* means "royal," and the meditation route to Self-Realization is considered to be just this. It is

Yoga and Yogic Science

direct and affords the opportunity of experience in different levels of awareness, beginning from where we start to where we are able to conclude after our meditation practice.

There are those new to the practice of Yoga who despair at ever being able to meditate. Only two things can prevent success in meditation: first, lack of understanding regarding the process; second, lack of will or resolution to meditate. Many persons today are given instruction in meditation without preliminary instruction regarding the prerequisites. Therefore, they do not have the necessary foundation upon which to build. Patanjali clearly defines the steps in the *Raja Yoga* system and insists upon full attention to every detail. I have covered this thoroughly in my book, *This is Reality*, a commentary of the *Yoga Sutras*, but let me summarize:

Raja Yoga meditation is the process whereby the yogin concentrates upon one point in order to integrate discontinuous, diffused attention, thus holding attention steady. All distractions are thus effectively closed out, and meditation proceeds. Daydreaming, floating with thoughts or allowing impulses to dominate is obviously not concentration, and, without concentration, meditation is impossible to experience. *Raja Yoga* is also known as "Eight-Limbed Yoga" or *Ashtanga Yoga*, because eight steps are prescribed.

1. Restraints (*yama*) are prescribed. These are: harmlessness (*ahimsa*)—not to injure any creature or any person in any way whatsoever; truthfulness (*satya*)—to be established in truth consciousness and to maintain this in all relationships; non-stealing (*asteya*)—to refrain from taking that which is not ours by right of Consciousness and *karma*; sense-control (*brahmacharya*)—to regulate the impulses and conserve energy, as well as to avoid complications; neutralizing the desire to acquire and hoard wealth (*aparigraha*), i.e.,—not to receive or have anything. These are the moral virtues which, if attended to, purify human nature and contribute to health and happiness of society. Most of these

restraints are obvious in their purpose and value. Two of them, *brahmacharya* and non-receiving, perhaps need a more extensive explanation. *Brahmacharya* is frequently defined as celibacy, and this is often recommended for Yoga students during either short periods of intense study and meditation or, later, when working with *kundalini*, for the purpose of transcending subtle levels of mind and consciousness. A more thorough discussion will follow later. Non-receiving means truly to renounce the desire to acquire things for the sake of false security, pride or vanity. There is obviously nothing wrong in a person's making wise use of things. It is obsession with things which is counseled against for the person who would be successful in the practice of Yoga.

2. The observances or disciplines (*niyama*) are: cleanliness (*śauca*), purification of body and organs of the body; serenity (*samtosa*), to be at peace within and content with one's lifestyle; asceticism (*tapas*), to confront and handle the inner urges without outer show, to be centered and non-reactive to the dualities, to burn out unwanted and destructive tendencies; study of the scriptures explaining the science of Yoga and Metaphysics (*Swadhyaya*) in order to be informed and motivated; and contemplation on God (*Īsvara*) in order to become attuned to God and God's will. A complete examination of human tendencies and characteristics is made in the *Yoga Sutras*, with suggestions for overcoming unwanted tendencies and developing desirable ones.

3. Yogic postures (*asanas*) are prescribed for the purpose of comfort and firmness during meditation and the practice of pranayamas. An upright seated posture in which one can sit with comfort and no need to move is ideal for meditation.

4. *Pranayama* gives control of breathing processes and control of vital force. When the inflowing breath is neutralized or joined with the outflowing breath, then perfect relaxation and balance of body activities are realized. In *Raja Yoga*, we are mainly concerned with balancing the flows of vital forces, then directing them

inward to the *chakra* system and upward to the crown *shakra* or thousand petaled lotus (*sahasara*).

5. When the senses are no longer tied to external sources, the result is restraint, interiorization or *pratyahara*. Now that the vital forces are flowing back to the Source within, one can concentrate without being distracted by externals or the temptation to cognize externals. A person experiences this state, to a degree, just before going to sleep or upon awakening. One is then aware but settled and not strongly impelled towards sense contact with the outer world. It is easy for us to "be in the world but not of it" when we learn to practice interiorization of the sense currents. We can be aware of the world (at times other than during meditation) but not be attached to it. Practicing this restraint, one soon finds that tendencies and habits are neutralized, because "needs" are abandoned.

6. Pure concentration (*dharana*) is the stage which follows. The attention is now fully directed to one point, whatever the yogi has chosen for this purpose: one of the *chakras*, the third eye, the crown *chakra*, a personal *mantra*, an attribute of God or the formless Reality. When no inner tendency obstructs, then concentration is pure or one-pointed.

7. Yogic meditation (*dhyana*) is perfect contemplation: concentration upon a point of focus with the intention of knowing the truth about it. Obviously, to flow the attention to one point will not result in insight or realization; one must identify and become "one with" the object of contemplation, in order to know for certain the truth about it.

8. *Samadhi* is the final stage in this Eight-Limbed Yoga. There are various stages of *samadhi*, depending upon whether one is identified with the object while yet conscious of the object, or whether one has transcended the object of meditation and is resting in the experience of being, without conceptual support or without support of any aspect of Consciousness.

Success in *Raja Yoga* practice calls for courage,

energy and high resolve. It is too easy for a person with weak resolve to be content with peace and relaxation as the fruits of meditation. The roots of the senses are in the mind; therefore, in deep meditation the senses are turned in upon themselves and abide in themselves. The next step is for one to extricate Consciousness from the organs of senses and the mind and to rest in the Transcendental Experience. This is *samadhi* without support. As long as one is identified with subtle senses in the mind, one can be brought into contact with the counterparts, the body senses and contact with the environment. In *samadhi*, one has closed the doors to sense identification and can rest in the experience realized. Simply because one experiences a state of *samadhi*, he is not necessarily liberated. One may experience identification with light, joy, sound or any object of concentration and still retain seeds of possible future problems in mind and consciousness. But such *samadhi* experiences can have a purifying and weakening effect upon the impressions of the mind. As long as one "enjoys" *samadhi*, there is the temptation to let enjoyment keep one from moving through the experience to knowledge. In some *samadhi* states, a yogi will experience Cosmic Consciousness, enter into astral or mental realms, or even temporarily lose the sense of individuality while absorbed in the meditation ideal. But, if upon returning to sense awareness, he loses the awareness of *samadhi*, his *samadhi* is not perfect or permanent.

The ideal is conscious awareness of the truth about life and about one's changeless nature at all times, whether meditating or not. This is *sahaja samadhi*, the natural, spontaneous awareness. When concentration, contemplation and *samadhi* are easy and natural, the result is called *samyama*, or the coming together of these stages. Then, by practicing in this manner relative to any object of focus, the yogi can easily gain realization and insight into the object to which he directs his attention. He can want to know, for instance, how the universe was formed and, by contemplating this, gain insight into the process. He can examine the scriptures with the intention to know the truth behind the words and to acquire esoteric insight. He can think of a person and know all about that person. Nothing is hidden from the person who has mastered concentration, contemplation and *samadhi*. And, in so far as he works in harmony with natural laws, nothing is impossible to him.

There is nothing wrong with using natural abilities to understand ourselves, others, the world process and the nature of God. What matters is the purity of mind and intention. This is why the first two steps in *Raja Yoga*, the restraints and the observances, are so important. One who is not pure in mind and intention can, with the advanced abilities acquired through Yoga, create serious problems for himself and others. The teaching is that as long as one is still striving for Self-Realization and liberation of consciousness, he should devote the better part of his time and energy to this end, rather than becoming too preoccupied with externals or the unfoldment of yogic powers. Many Yoga teachers stress that the powers (*siddhis*) should not be sought, they should be allowed to unfold. As long as a person is seeking these powers, he is still in ego consciousness and can not be trusted with them if he does acquire them.

The *siddhis* are referred to as "miraculous powers," at least from the point of view of one who does not understand or have them. One can master the elements by truly understanding them. Some of the *siddhis* are: knowing previous life-cycles by contemplating the residue of subconscious impressions of self or others; tuning in to the mental states of others and knowing their thoughts; contemplating an atom and being one with the atom; being one with the universe; obtaining anything desired; controlling the elements and natural forces; satisfying desire by an act of will—even materializing things by an act of will; overcoming time by flowing attention back to the source of time and many others. I want to emphasize that these claims are not extreme ones, they are all within the realm of experience.

A master of Yoga will only use *siddhis* after being sure, through intuitive guidance, that his use of yogic ability will be of value to those involved and to the evolutionary process. There are some yogis who refuse to exert any will power at all, but they rest in the natural state of God-Realization and let whatever happens just happen. Healings, intervention in problem situations, spiritual awakening of disciples and other occurrences are reported because of one's attunement with a master of Yoga. Such a master, if pressed, will deny any personal will or effort in relationship to the happenings. Immersed in God Consciousness he might simply say, "It is all God's will."

There are other yogic systems mentioned here and there, but they are really only a matter of emphasis. The basic philosophy and procedures are being included in the systems reviewed here. In the *Bhagavad-Gita*, Krishna instructs Arjuna regarding the characteristics to be found in the ideal yogi. The opening verses of chapter sixteen explain:

"Courage, purity of mind, wise use of knowledge, concentration, generosity, self-control and right use of abilities, along with faithful study of scriptures and noble purpose; non-violence, truth, freedom from anger, renunciation, tranquility, freedom from finding fault, compassion and faithfulness, vigor, forgiveness, persistence, selflessness, freedom from the desire to harm others, and freedom from excessive pride; these are the natural endowments of a person who is born with a divine nature."

It is not expected that all persons will be born with these natural inclinations so desirable for success in life and on the spiritual path. This is why we have Yoga and the disciplines of training. No matter what the present condition of a person, if he will but prepare himself and begin on a wise course of action, he will, in time, be successful in his venture.

Chapter Two
THE NATURE OF THE WORLD
and STAGES OF SELF-REALIZATION

Since the goal of one on the spiritual path is Enlightenment, we shall examine the nature and characteristics of Consciousness in order to obtain some understanding regarding exactly what an enlightened person comes to know directly. There is, of course, a difference between knowing about a thing versus knowing a thing by experiencing it. As my param-guru, Sri Yukteswar, often said, "Wisdom is not assimilated with the eyes, but with the atoms." Belief may precede knowledge, but knowledge of a thing alone allows total understanding. I may believe something but not fully understand it. Therefore, belief in the usefulness of spiritual disciplines and faith that we shall experience the ultimate realization can be a prerequisite to final success or Enlightenment.

While teachers and enlightened persons (who play the role of teacher to those whose interest is improved function but not Self-Realization) will usually advise along general lines for the peace and well-being of individuals and society, a true master of Yoga is ever alert for that special seeker who has the innate potential for liberation of consciousness in this incarnation. This liberation is the result of the soul's awakening to a clear insight regarding the nature of Supreme Consciousness, God, and the world process. The experience, the way to the experience and the explanation of the nature of the life process are one. *Darsana* is not only the philosophy but also the approach to understanding and the understanding (direct perception) itself. Then things are seen and known in true perspective. The way and the experience is known as the Holy Science or *Kaivalya Darsana*. One thereby knows the characteristics of this world as well as That which is the Cause and Support of it. In the words of Jesus: "And you shall know the truth, and the truth shall make you free."

The motivation of persons on the spiritual path can be mild or intense. That is, one might be inclined toward Self-Realization but not to the extent of doing much about it. One might be more disciplined but still caught between the urge for knowledge, on the one hand, and the desire for human satisfaction on the other. Or one might be totally dedicated to the philosophy and the practice of Yoga. The progress of a person will be equal to the motivation and the practice. One who, himself, is not yet fully self-realized can be a teacher to seekers whose motivations are mild or moderate in intensity, for he can share what he knows and thus encourage the student on the path. One who is intense on the path and whose goal is liberation of consciousness will require a *Sat-Guru*, an illumined guru who knows the way and is himself fully enlightened. We cannot teach another that which we do not know, and we cannot impart to another that which we do not possess. The *Sat-Guru* is an incarnation of pure knowledge and realization. All *Sat-Gurus* teach the same basic message, because they see the true order of things. The superficial teachings regarding social manners and religious worship will differ according to time, place (cultural setting) and individual and group needs, but the underlying message regarding the nature of the world process, the Reality of the soul and the way to Enlightenment will always be the same. A seeker who is looking for a different, unique, novel or special philosophy is not a sincere truth seeker. The ideal for one who is dedicated to Yoga-Darsana is to embark humbly upon a program of study, practice and experience which leads to knowledge.

The Essential Truth

Here, then, is the teaching regarding the nature of

The Nature of the World 31

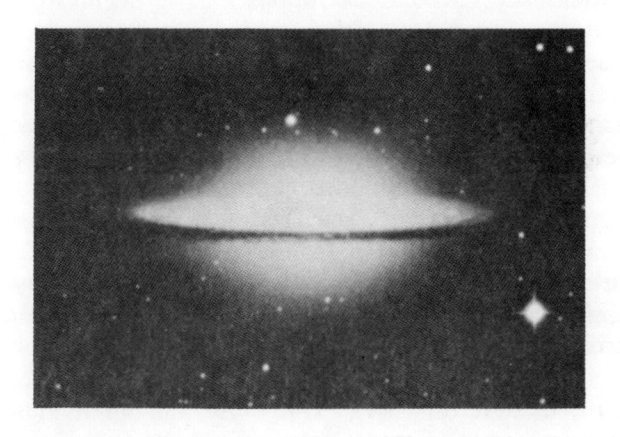

the world process. *Supreme Consciousness (Spirit, Reality, Consciousness) is the only thing there is, from subtle to gross levels of expression, and there is nothing else.* Until we are intuitively and intellectually awakened, we cannot comprehend the subtle side of nature. We can, with sense perception only, perceive the outer side or the world of effects. By acquiring inner vision, we can also perceive the world of cause and, in this way, know the total story. This is why it is taught that man who is limited to mind and to sense perception cannot comprehend the nature of Ultimate Reality. For this, he must be "born again" or possessed of soul perception. Because we have an intuitive knowing regarding the truth of this philosophy as expounded by the seers, we can have faith, we can hope for knowledge, and we can eventually awaken to the truth. When Jesus taught: "When you have lifted up the son of man, then shall you know I am he," he spoke the truth. When we are able to raise our consciousness, elevate our point of view above the limitations of mind and senses, we can see clearly that the soul is truly a ray of Supreme Consciousness reflecting in the medium of the mind. When we assume ourselves to be mind (*manas*), we are man; when we know ourselves as a reflection of Supreme Consciousness working through the mind, we are seeing from the level of Self-Realization.

Supreme Consciousness, the absolute, non-dual aspect of Consciousness, is without attributes or characteristics. It just is; It remains ever the same. When attributes and qualities emerge on the screen of time and space (which are themselves the product of Supreme Consciousness), we then are able to analyze, examine, relate to, and understand this outer expression of Consciousness. The absolute non-dual aspect can be experienced but not examined. God is that aspect of Supreme Consciousness which first appears as It begins to flow into manifestation. God is, therefore, Supreme Consciousness in the initial out-picturing process. We do not refer to Supreme Consciousness *and* God, any more than we refer to God *and* the world. We refer to Supreme Consciousness *as* God and *as* the world process. We also refer to Supreme Consciousness *as* the soul. Shankara, the great philosopher-sage, in his explanation regarding the nature of Consciousness, explained that the soul is a reflection of Supreme Consciousness shining in the organ of intelligence (the discerning aspect of the mind).

In other words, we practice our disciplines in order to disentangle ourselves from body and mind identification, so that we can clearly recall our true nature as Supreme Consciousness. This is the purpose of *Yoga-Darsana*. This is important to remember, for there are many who are involved with the practice of Yoga who make the practice the end, instead of awakening fully to the realization of the truth. Preliminary Yogas give

The Nature of the World

mastery of body and mind: *Raja Yoga* gives the experience of the soul nature and aspects of Consciousness, including the experience of Pure Consciousness; *Jnana Yoga* brings direct knowledge (and experience) through the process of discernment.

In God are the qualities of *being, consciousness-intelligence and creative energy*. As we are what God is, a reflection of Supreme Consciousness, we likewise possess the qualities of *being, consciousness-intelligence and creative energy*. This is why all authentic scriptures declare man to be made in the image and likeness of God. This is why Self or Soul-Realization results in God-Realization. By directing attention inwardly, a person can cognize the qualities of his own nature and know himself as a divine expression. The quality of being enables us to know ourselves as immortal, changeless Reality; the quality of consciousness-intelligence enables us to be aware and to know; the quality of creative energy enables us to will and to do. A person is not God and never will be, but a person is a godlike-being who can relate to God and work in harmony with God's will.

When the Creative Energy of God expresses as outflowing force balanced with the attracting aspect of the Being quality, a vibration results, which is discerned as the Word: *Amen, OM, Aum, Pranava*. As this Current flows out in the direction of manifestation, It gives rise to the characteristics of time (*kala*), space (*desa*) and particles or atoms (*patra* or *anu*). These along with the current Itself make up the four aspects of the Word and make it possible for God to appear as the world process. The Word then becomes flesh or appears as the outer universe. The Word, being a manifestation of God, is inseparable from God and is God. *John 1:1-3 and 14* explains this in the same way: "In the beginning was the Word, and the Word was with God, and the Word was God . . . all things were made by Him; and without Him was not anything made that was made . . . and the Word was made flesh and dwelt among us." When the yogi attunes his attention to the internal sound of OM, the sound of the creative energy within, he can follow this stream of sound back to the Source or soul-nature.

The particles or atoms taken together are referred to as the Throne of Spirit, because Spirit shining on them and reflecting in them makes possible the world process. Atoms (or particles), flowing creative energy, time and space (all considered as one basic fabric) are referred to as the substance of which all outer things are formed. This fabric or basic stuff of nature is also referred to as *maya*, The Darkness, because one who is identified with this substance and forgetful (or unaware) of the cause and nature of that which produced it out of Itself is not able to comprehend the true order of things. He is, therefore, ignorant of the truth about life. Being deluded or spiritually unaware, a person who desires liberation is in need of spiritual quickening and awakening. Through the practice of certain disciplines, one learns to see through the appearance-world and comprehends the nature of Consciousness both within and without. He is then firm in knowledge and has overcome the world.

The current of repulsion gives rise to the fabric which makes possible the manifestation of the gross world. Again, this fabric is the sound current, out of which evolves time, space and the particles or atoms. The attracting aspect of the Godhead shines on this fabric (*maya*) and, in time, redeems it—that is, draws it back to the Source from which it originally began. The life-awakening and Consciousness-awakening attracting aspect vitalizing nature is referred to as the Holy Spirit. God as the outflowing current appears as the stuff of the world, and God as the attracting aspect awakens dormant vitality and draws it back to the point of origin. Individualizations of Spirit, awakening through forms of matter, are referred to as Sons of God. In every form of matter there is life and the potential for awakening. This is why evolution takes place and why

The Nature of the World

the world process is flowing towards the point of origin.

A polarized ray of Supreme Consciousness attracts to itself a magnetic aura, the initial subtle vehicle or sheath through which it expresses in the outer realm. Under the influence of the attracting aspect, the Holy Spirit, the part of this magnetic field in which Supreme Consciousness can be self-cognized is known as the Intelligence (*Buddhi*); the opposite polarity of this magnetic field is known as mind (*manas*). When identified with Intelligence, the individualization of Supreme Consciousness is known as Supreme Consciousness-with-identification (Atman). When identified with the mind aspect, this individualization of Supreme Consciousness is known as soul (*jiva*). When established in discernment (Intelligence), one is liberated; when identified with mind, one is in bondage and in need of being "saved" or awakened. Furthermore, when the ray of Supreme Consciousness is possessed of consciousness (awareness) while identified with mind, it also has feeling. The deepest feeling of which we are capable is that of feeling our nature as being. Because of involvement with mind through feeling, the sense of separate existence is felt: this is ego (*ahamkara*). Thus, the Son of God becomes the son of man (mind or *manas*). By awakening to the realization of our basic nature, we shift our viewpoint from being a limited human being to knowing ourself as an unlimited divine being. Because we are truly divine, we can recall this essential nature. By removing the restricting characteristics from mind and the other sheaths or coverings of the true nature, we consciously realize who and what we are.

The faculty of intelligence is used, by those seeking Self-Realization, to discern clearly the truth about the nature of Consciousness. The mind aspect is used to relate to the world, to set and reach goals and to experience pleasurable sensations. The outflowing tendency of Creative Energy, when identified with the mind, is the cause of desire, which leads toward fulfillment of desire through the senses. When the current is made to flow back to the Source in the practice of meditation and calm self-analysis, the outflowing tendency is neutralized, and one then is able to live in the world without attachment or strong sensual urges. We experience through the senses when relating to the world, but we do so with understanding and self-control, once we are established in Yoga.

At the level of God-mind or Universal Mind, the outflowing current through *maya* appears as the world process. The outer world is cognized by the soul through the five senses. With intuition and the subtle senses, the yogi is able to cognize the finer realm which supports and nourishes the gross world.

Individualized polarized Supreme Consciousness (*jiva* or soul) extends into five aura electricities, which make up the causal sheath or vehicle of the soul. These five electricities (*pancha tattwa*) produce the organs of sense (*jnanandriyas*), organs of action (*karmendrivas*) and the objects of the senses (*tanmatras*). This happens because of the influence of the three natural attributes (*gunas*) which are respectively: positive (*sattwa*), neutralizing (*rajas*) and negative (*tamas*). These fifteen attributes, along with mind and intelligence, constitute the seventeen subtle aspects of the spiritual body (*lingasarira*). In this subtle body are the counterparts later to be reflected in the gross physical form, and the five electricities are referred to as root-causes. It is with this subtle body that the soul moves through inner planes, when absent from the physical form.

The organs of sense are smell, taste, sight, touch and hearing. The neutralizing attributes of the five electricities result in the organs of action: excretion, generation, speech, motion and manual skill. The organs of sense are rooted in the mind. The organs of action are rooted in a body of energy. The negative attributes of the five electricities enable one to experience temporary satisfaction as a result of fulfilling desire through the senses. They are also the cause of the production of the physical form comprised of solids (*kshiti*), liquids (*ap*), fire (*tejas*), gaseous substances or air (*marut*), and ether (*akasa*) or fine matter. Combinations of subtle elements result in the appearance of gross matters, and the physical world is produced. From the Godhead to fully physical manifestation, *prana* flows and, by a process of self-modification, appears as all that is beheld.

The gross elements of the physical realm, along with the fifteen subtle attributes, mind, feeling, ego sense and intelligence make up the twenty-four principles underlying the entire phenomenal universe. St. John discerned this in deep meditation as set forth in *Revelation 4:4*, "And round about the throne were four and twenty seats; and upon the seats I saw four and twenty elders (electric principles)." Because of these principle aspects of Consciousness, the world drama is possible. This is why sages declare that the life process is a play of Consciousness. The creative energy making possible this process is known as *shakti*, female energy producing and nourishing all forms.

Furthermore, the universe is a series of fourteen spheres, seven levels of descending manifestation (*lokas*) and seven corresponding *chakras*, distribution points through which current flows to nourish and sustain the manifest realms. In descending order these levels are described as:

a. The sphere of God and the level where God-Realized souls dwell. This is known as *Satyaloka*, the sphere of truth consciousness. Here souls experience constant *samadhi* and are not involved with externals.

b. The sphere of the Holy Spirit, *Tapoloka*, where souls are also absorbed in bliss consciousness.

c. The sphere of spiritual reflection, where souls have a sense of separate existence but are highly self-realized. This is *Janaloka*, where radiant beings dwell in glory and spiritual power.

d. The sphere where *maya* appears and the outer worlds begin to manifest. This is *Maharloka*, the connecting place between the subtle realms and the material universe. Moving through this level, the gods take on bodies of matter and, moving from the realm of matter to the subtle spheres, they leave the outer realm behind. This is refered to as the door (*Dasamadwara*) between the inner and the outer realms.

  e. The sphere of magnetic auras or electricities, which is *Swarloka*, beyond the level of gross matter, as well as of subtle matter.

  f. The sphere of electric attributes, *Bhuvarloka*, the realm of fine matters which precede the next sphere in order of manifestation. Here is the astral realm.

  g. The sphere of gross material manifestation, *Bhuloka*, which is cognized through the senses.

The spheres flow out of the Godhead. Since the soul is made in the image and the likeness of God, vital force flows from it to appear as the corresponding sheaths or vehicles and works through vital centers, which are the *chakras*. By ascending through the *chakras*, a person can awaken to the knowledge of the corresponding spheres of creation and gain access to the realm of God. When current flows down through the *chakras*, the soul is bound to the body. When the current ascends, transformation of the body is effected, and Self-Realization is experienced. The descending current forms the body, and the ascending current transforms it. Only a small portion of the available energy is used by the average person; the major part remains dormant as *kundalini* (dormant potential). Prayer, meditation, relaxation, chanting and the grace of God stirs *kundalini* and encourages it to ascend. *Shaktipat* initiation at the hands of a *Sat-Guru* is also a powerful influence. *Pranayamas* and *mudras* aid in the process of awakening and transformation.

The divine nature is said to be screened by five sheaths (koshas) or coverings. The first sheath is the polarized particle of Supreme Consciousness, which becomes mildly identified with *maya*. This is the seat of feeling (*chitta*), sometimes referred to as one's heart. When a *guru* tells the disciple to "seek out the truth in the heart," he is referring to an analysis of this most subtle part of the inner nature and not to any *chakra* or physical organ. The second screen or sheath is the organ of intelligence, which is formed by the action of the positive polarity on the magnetic aura. Use of this organ enables one to have true knowledge through discernment. The third sheath is the mind, composed of the organs of the senses. The fourth sheath is the astral or vital body. The fifth is the physical body. In order, these are named according to their nature as: *anandamaya kosha* (bliss sheath); *jnanamaya kosha* (knowledge sheath); *manomaya kosha* (mind sheath); *pranamaya kosha* (vital force sheath); and *annamaya kosha* (food sheath), which is sustained by material nourishment.

When the worlds are fully extended or manifested, the action of the attracting pole of the Godhead begins to draw energies back to the point of origin. In this manner, life appears on planets and life forms evolve as Consciousness awakens and makes the return to God. In reference to a person who is spiritually awakening, this process continues from gross to subtle levels. When one awakens sufficiently to realize he is more than a body, he becomes aware of the vital energies which sustain the body. He is then ready to practice Yoga and to work with the currents which flow through the system. Directing them intelligently, he quickens his own spiritual evolution rather than remaining at the mercy of natural influences, such as fresh air, sunlight, nourishing food, planetary energies and the trends of nature. This is why Yoga is for our current time cycle, as well as for one in any time cycle who has sufficiently awakened to the level of grasping the usefulness of the discipline.

As one's attention is drawn to the awareness of subtle levels, one experiences greater awareness and freedom and can more easily understand the workings of natural laws, as seen in the material environment. After the worlds are formed, dormant vital force begins to withdraw from matter. As it withdraws from the material sheath, *prana* becomes more pronounced and plants appear. As it withdraws from the vital sheath, animals appear. As it withdraws from the mind sheath, man appears. When man is able to become aware of his inmost nature, he becomes luminous and self-realized. When the self-realized person withdraws from identification with the feeling nature and the aura electricities, he becomes supremely free, a Son of God, and merges into the pure light of Spirit. In this sequence does the involved Supreme Consciousness return to the Source or to the condition existing prior to manifestation.

When a person arrives at the level of understanding where he intellectually comprehends that the outer world is really a reflection or extension of a finer cause, he begins his move in consciousness to higher realization. He is then ready for initiation, either from a *Sat-Guru* or through the inner soul-process, which is the equivalent of the outer *guru*. In most instances, because one newly awakened to the prospect of higher knowledge is not yet possessed of keen intuition and sharp discernment, the Intelligence of God will come into his life as a true *guru*. By receiving the flow of energy (grace) from the *guru* and by receiving practical instruction, a devoted person makes rapid progress on the path of Yoga. In due time, the aspirant becomes aware of the inner sound current and is able to follow it to the point of origin, where he then experiences the clear state. In many religious teachings, this sound current is referred to as a river over which one can cross to reach the promised land or idealized sphere of consciousness. For instance, Christians speak of crossing over the Jordan river, and Hindus have faith in the river Ganges as a purifying influence.

Being baptized and immersed in the sound current, one is "born of the Spirit." Without this second birth, there is no chance of spiritual progress, for one will remain sense-bound and sense-oriented. Here one repents or turns the attention back to the source of origin. In time, the seeker who is steady on the path overcomes restrictions of matter and comprehends the inner realms, the nature of *maya* and the true nature of God. Liberation (*Kaivalya*) is the result of total Self-Realization: here one realizes there is no separate self—that Supreme Consciousness is the only Reality and is appearing as Everything involved in the cosmic drama. Devotion to the highest ideal and love of God results in a magnetic attraction that hastens the liberation experience.

When all of the conditionings are removed from the subtle nature, then one no longer reflects the light of Spirit but actually manifests this light. One is thus annointed with Christ Consciousness (the Intelligence-governing aspect of the Godhead) and, if still working within the framework of time and space, plays the role of savior or *Sat-Guru* to others. Not only is this soul's liberation assured, but, through such a one, the Divine Power also works for the liberation of others, when they are receptive to the influence.

Yoganandaji was fond of quoting *John 1:12*: "But as many as received him, to them gave he power to become the Sons of God, even to them that believe (commune) on his name." The name is the Word, the sound current which flows from the Godhead. By communing with this current, one's attention flows to God. Comprehending himself as seeming-individualized consciousness floating in the light of OM, the renunciate then abandons the idea of separate existence and awakens to the experience of Oneness. This return in understanding to the Source is called permanent liberation.

Liberation as the Ideal of Yoga

A person begins to yearn for liberation when he begins to realize that the outer realms have to do with relativities and forever change. Liberation is described as that state wherein one is stabilized in Self-Realization. He is, therefore, no longer in bondage due to the influences of nature and can experience no further pain. Identified with the forever-becomingness (*samsara*) of this and other worlds, the soul is destined to continue blind movement through time and space. Exponents of *Jnana Yoga* teach that human problems are basically due to false assumptions about that which is not permanent and to lack of perception of that which is Real or changeless. When a person takes the material world to be the only reality, he is, of course, doomed to suffer the consequences of such misunderstanding. There is a word for ignorance in this philosophical treatise, in keeping with the tradition of careful and precise analysis of Consciousness manifesting, and that word is *avidya*, ignorance of what is true. Inherent in *maya* is *avidya*, ignorance. Being polarized, it manifests as egoism, attachment, aversion and blind identification. The darkening power (*tamas*) of *maya* produces egoism and identification; the polarity influence of *maya* produces attachment through attraction and aversion, as a result of repulsion. Thus, a person under the spell of *maya* tends either to be attracted to nature or to be repelled by it, instead of being centered and viewing the cosmic process with understanding. One may feel that, by becoming attached to the object of attraction, happiness will be realized, and, by avoiding contact with that which is repulsive, pain will be avoided. Persistent identification with outer realms is due to the fact that the person so identified feels the outer realms to be the only real ones. One clings to that which is assumed to be real or permanent. Immersed in *maya*, the fabric of nature, one is deluded and attached and plays the role of an unknowing participant.

Every master has taught the same basic truth: the cause of suffering is ignorance (of the true nature of things); the solution to the problem is Enlightenment. All spiritual disciplines and recommendations are designed to enable a person to awaken and to see things in proper perspective. Disciplines cannot cause liberation of consciousness, but, by affording the opportunity for clearing the mind and purifying the sheaths, the disciplines can allow the light of the soul to shine in brilliance and glory.

We suffer because, being identified with *maya*, we act from the basis of egoism, thus making mistakes. If we are wise, we learn to live in harmony with the universe, thereby avoiding mistakes and the consequent pain and frustration they bring in their wake. We are naturally (not always *usually*) inclined towards the conscious experience of being, awareness and bliss—these being the characteristics of our nature as Supreme Consciousness. Bliss does not refer to happiness or joy but to the serene awareness of feeling while purely conscious. Our drive for fleeting joys and pleasurable experiences springs from our unconscious urge to experience the bliss of soul awareness. We learn, through study and experience, to direct the attention and the life currents within so that the desire for fulfillment can be neutralized and balanced internally. In this manner, we learn that fulfillment is never to be had on a permanent, unchanging basis in the outer world. When one is able to satisfy the urge for fulfillment by turning within and experiencing the real nature, he becomes contented. A sense-driven person can never know lasting contentment, nor can a person know contentment who suppresses natural desires in order to avoid involvement and pain. Only when the currents are balanced and the inner realization is clear and stable can one be at peace. This is why it is taught that the kingdom of heaven or fulfillment is within. With contentment, one can be stable on the spiritual path and devote time to constructive work in the world without ego involvement, and time to meditation, without personal desire for phenomenal results and happenings. Total surrender and renunciation of personal ambition is required of one who would be absorbed in the stream of light which accompanies the inner sound current. In due time, one awakens from the sense of limitation and realizes his own nature as the indestructible Self or Supreme Consciousness. This final state is not Oneness-with God: it is *Oneness*.

The Way to the Ideal

Here is the most direct route to Self-Realization: self-discipline and self-purification (*tapas*); deep, contemplative study of truth principles (*swadhyaya*); and meditation on Om (*Brahmanidhana*). To be self-disciplined, one must do what must be done to succeed in a venture, avoid that which is non-productive and be patient and non-reactive at all times. Contemplative study means to read, analyze and perceive the truth of that which is studied. The final step is to merge consciously in the Word, the sound current. OM (*Aum, Amen*) is the primal sound, the sound heard when all other sounds have subsided. Merging with (not merely listening to) the sound current is possible when we are devoted to God, possessed of courage and will to go all the way, capable of "remembering" the truth regarding our real condition, and resulting when perfect in *samadhi*. When we love God and the spiritual ideal, we are encouraged to persist in spite of temporary obstacles and setbacks. Without courage, little of any real value can be accomplished in the outer or the inner worlds. Floating in the sound, while a useful relaxation practice, will not lead to Enlightenment. There must be the flow of attention to the Source, if the transcendental experience is to be had.

All people who are not awakened, and who desire to be, need some ideal upon which to focus. Some persons worship aspects of nature, others worship a human ideal. Clear minded persons worship the Divine Light. At whatever level we begin, we can wholeheartedly become involved, always remembering to give up the lower for the higher, when the higher realization is experienced. We differ in capacity and ability; therefore, we worship the ideal which seems most real and useful for our focus.

To assure steadiness on the path and to afford the opportunity for clearing mind and consciousness, the yogi is encouraged to observe basic guidelines or reli-

The Nature of the World

gious rules. The recommendations of all the prophets, in so far as they are universal in application, are given for the purpose of easing man's journey in this world and insuring harmony with others and nature. In the *Yoga Sutras*, the student is specifically instructed to abide by the observances known as *yama* and *niyama*, which have been explained in the preceding chapter. By observing the guidelines, being natural in lifestyle and attentive to disciplines of yoga and meditation practice, one quickly alters the course of human destiny and attains Realization.

This, in brief, is the view of life-as-consciousness as seen by seers possessed of inner vision. This philosphical treatise is not a belief-system. It is simply an explanation of what is seen when soul perception is clear and the cosmic processes are understood. Furthermore, the teachings of the masters is that all souls will one day awaken to the truth about the nature of the life process. Whether one on the path awakens quickly or slowly depends on a number of conditions: the innate capacity when the quest is started; the will to see it through and do what has to be done; and the grace of God. My *guru* told me that a person is not even drawn to the path of yoga unless he is ready for the discipline involved. We have the power of choice as to whether or not we will take up the challenge and the opportunity which lies before us, once the way has been made clear.

Chapter Three
PURIFICATION OF THE BODY

Leaving nothing to chance, the masters of Yoga explain that a person who would be perfected in Yoga must see to the basic requirements, which are seven in number: body purification, strength of mind and body, steadfastness, patience, lightness of body, direct perception and transcendence of the world.

Purification of the body is recommended first. If the body is healthy and functional, the mind will also function properly, and one will be able to proceed without illness or difficulty from this level.

The practice of *Yogasanas* (Yoga poses) insures strength of body and gives mental control, because one must realize the relationship between body and mind to be able to practice the *asanas* correctly.

To be steadfast, one must be able to do whatever he determines to do until the goal is reached. *Mudras*, which give control over the involuntary nervous system, assist in this end.

Patience is a requirement, for change does not always come quickly. The practice of withdrawing attention and vital currents from the senses, through meditation, enables one to rest in a relaxed and settled condition and to be patient, while the inner work is being done and transformation takes place.

Lightness of the body is assured by the practice of *pranayamas* and attention to diet. *Pranayamas* cleanse the nerve pathways (*nadis*), and diet chosen for healthful purposes insures a disease free body.

Direct perception of the truth of that contemplated is attained by the practice of meditation and by the use of the faculty of intelligence.

World transcendence is the result of *samadhi*, where-

Purification of the Body

in one literally remains detached and unmoved regardless of what is perceived, because one is aware of the total cosmic picture.

Body Cleansing Processes

Daily cleansing of the body is recommended, washing thoroughly from head to feet to remove accumulated grime, oils and dead skin cells. Hair should be washed regularly, nails kept clean and trimmed, and good grooming habits developed. During the morning cleansing routine, one should clean the mouth-including tongue, gums and teeth. The modern practice of using dental floss to clean particles from between the teeth and below the gum line is recommended.

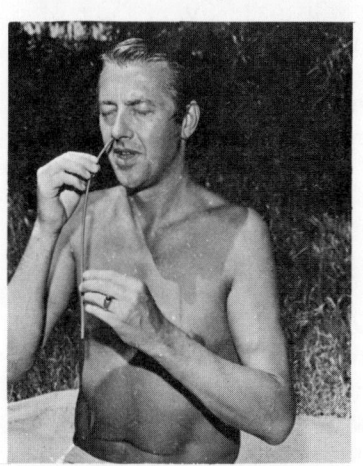

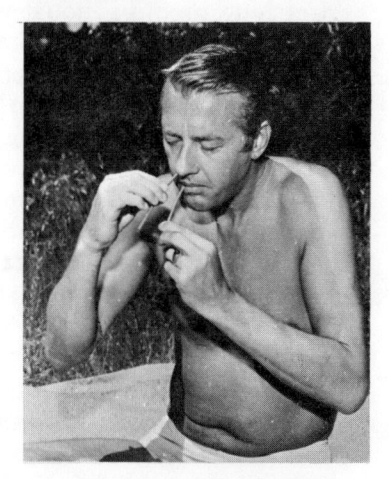

Nasal cleansing is a useful daily routine and can be accomplished in one or two ways—or both. If a rubber catheter can be obtained (a number 12 is a good size), one simply lubricates it and inserts it gently into the nasal passage until it is felt in the throat. Then one slowly removes it. This process is repeated with the other nostril. After this, take a shallow bowl full of warm water into which a pinch of salt has been stirred:

hold one nostril closed, *gently* suck water up the other nostril and expel it from the mouth into the sink. Repeat with the other nostril. This will wash mucus from the nasal passage quite effectively. Head cavities will be cleared of collected matter. Because of the proximity of the eyes, stimulation of the nasal passage with both the catheter and the water will influence nerves leading to the eyes and strengthen the eyes. It is also taught by yogis that, when the eyes are thus stimulated, a current flows back through the optic nerve to the brain, which has beneficial effects on glands in the head. For a more thorough use of the catheter, when it reaches the throat after insertion, pull it through the mouth, putting mild pressure against the soft palate. This will encourage a more complete cleansing of the head cavities, and the stretching of the soft palate will make the practice of *Kechari Mudra* (of which more will be written later) easier, when time comes to include this in the daily routine. Nasal cleansing can be done every morning for a period of time, then a few times a week as one feels the need or is so inclined.

Internal cleansing of the stomach and intestinal tract is recommended now and then, even if one is on a healthy diet. It should certainly be done if one is new at Yoga practices and wants to remove from the system the debris collected as a result of unwise eating and living habits. As the first liquid in the morning, take a glass of hot water, into which the juice of half a lemon has been squeezed, and drink it. This will encourage intestinal activity, act as a stimulant and provide a cleansing influence throughout the system. To cleanse the lower intestinal tract, use an enema: body temperature water (preferably distilled) can be taken into the system with the aid of an enema bag and rubber tube. Hold the water for as long as comfortable and then expel it from the body. If one is toxic, this cleansing process can be done a few days in a row. When on a short or long fast, take an enema daily to assist the body in throwing off waste which is being released from the system, the

Purification of the Body

organs and the tissues into the bowel. If the liver is sluggish and needs detoxification and stimulation, use a coffee enema: two to four tablespoons of regular grind coffee in a quart of water, made in the regular way; when down to body temperature, use as in the regular enema routine, retaining the water for ten to fifteen minutes before expelling.

For inner cleansing by fasting: mix the juice of six lemons, six grapefruits and twelve oranges in a gallon of distilled water. Whenever thirsty during the fast, drink until satisfied. Distilled water is useful, because the ions of distilled water have a positive electrical charge, which sucks collected salts and urea from the body tissues and carries them out in the urine.

After internal cleansing, if one will eat live foods in proper combinations and quantity, obtain sufficient exercise and remain free from stress and mental-emotional problems, the body will function efficiently and the mind will be clear and strong.

All of the *asanas, pranayamas* and *mudras* will be useful in that they encourage free circulation of vital forces, stimulate the glands, improve blood and lymphatic circulation, and release body wastes as well as mental-emotional blockages. It is through attention to internal and external cleansing and the techniques of Yoga that some Yoga masters are able to maintain a youthful body for decades longer than ordinary persons, if not for centuries.

A useful morning routine is to attend to body cleansing, then practice the Stomach Lift (*Uddiyana Bandha*) and other stomach exercises before *pranayama* and meditation.

Chapter Four
ASANAS FOR HEALTH AND MASTERY

There are literally dozens of *Yogasanas* or Yoga poses recommended in various ancient texts. There is little doubt but that the mastery of these poses is conducive to health and to increased awareness and function. It is not necessary for one to practice all of the asanas during one session. The usual program will include a series of complementary poses chosen to affect all areas of the body.

When practicing *Yogasanas*, one should be relaxed, wear few garments, be assured of a quiet and well ventilated room and proceed in a meditative mood. Remember, *Yogasanas* lead to *pranayama, mudra* and meditation; *Hatha Yoga* is preparation for *Raja Yoga*. Never should there be too much exertion, straining or working to the point of fatigue. One should always remain within the boundaries of personal capacity. It is not necessary for one to duplicate perfectly the poses as illustrated; the useful thing will be to assume them as nearly as one is able. By the practice of *Yogasanas*, the blood is circulated more completely throughout the system, lymphatic fluid is circulated, muscles are toned and strengthened, nerves are nourished, the flow of vital force is balanced, glands are stimulated and the bones of the body are placed in correct position. Extra benefits are increased energy, realization of the relationship between mind and body and self-confidence.

We usually practice asanas in a sequence that will afford a balancing effect on the muscular and the nervous systems. The grouping of poses as outlined here is designed to meet this end. If these poses are practiced upon awakening in the morning, the body is often too stiff for comfort and for ease of performance without warming up exercises. Later in the day, after the system has been in motion for a time, is usually a better occasion for practice. One will have to experiment to find what is most useful for personal practice. Allow at least thirty minutes for the practice of *asanas*. A blanket or mat on the floor will insure greater comfort.

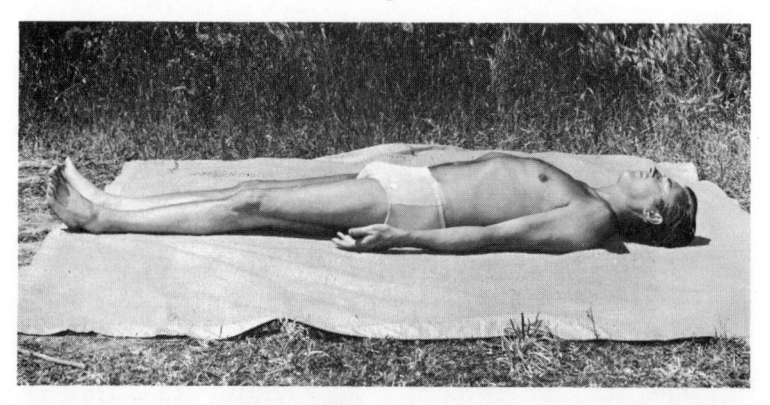

Corpse Pose (*Savasana*)

To be used between poses when convenient, the Corpse Pose allows total relaxation. Simply let the muscles relax, feel the circulation of *prana* throughout the system and be attuned to cosmic energies. This pose can also be practiced any time when one requires a few minutes of total rest and relaxation. If desired, one can watch the breathing rhythm and inwardly chant the *mantra* of one's choice.

Shoulder Stand (*Sarvangasana*)

The Shoulder Stand is one of the most refreshing of the *asanas*. This pose takes the strain off legs, rests the heart and stimulates thyroid gland function, while bringing a rich supply of blood to the brain and organs in the head cavity. Starting from the Corpse Pose, simply bring the lower part of the body slowly and gracefully back, until the full pose is accomplished. If one cannot assume the completed pose with ease, the modified position will do until flexibility is acquired. Hold for a few seconds or several seconds, if comfortable, and resume the Corpse Pose. Rest a few moments and repeat. Do this three to five times, resting and never straining between positions.

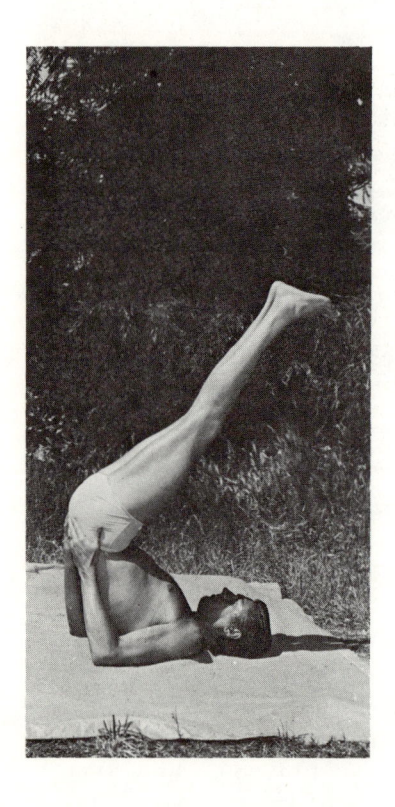

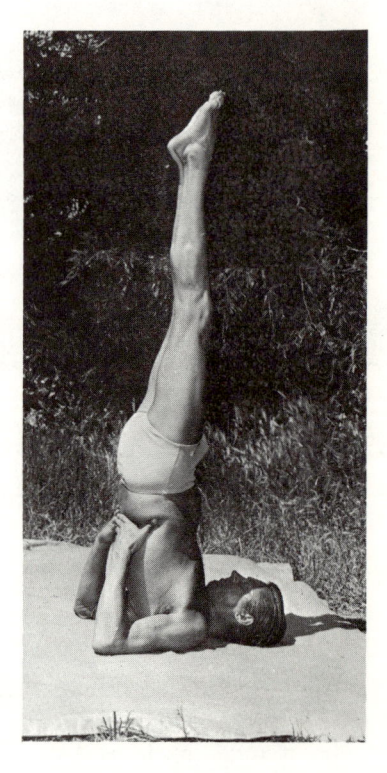

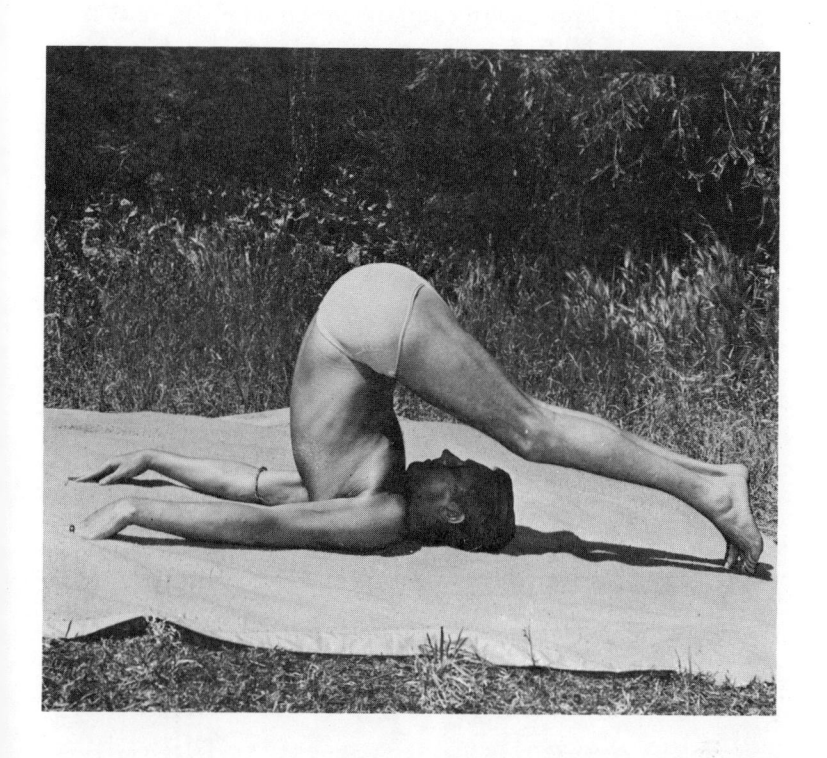

Plow Pose (*Halasana*)

This pose is a variation of the Shoulder Stand. When proficiency is attained in the Shoulder Stand, complete the Shoulder Stand series with the Plow Pose. This pose offers similar benefits to the Shoulder Stand and gives greater flexibility and strength to the upper body.

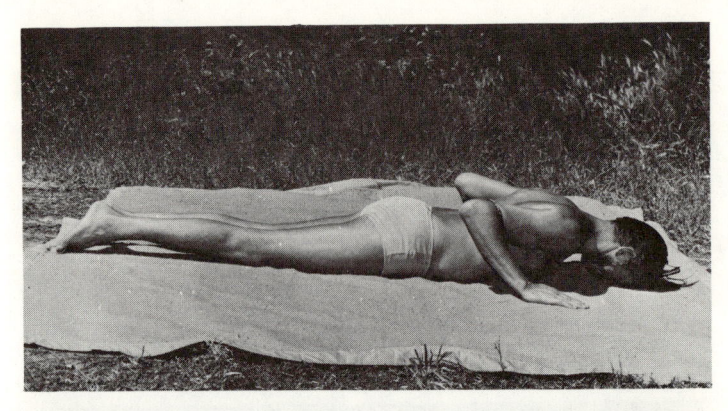

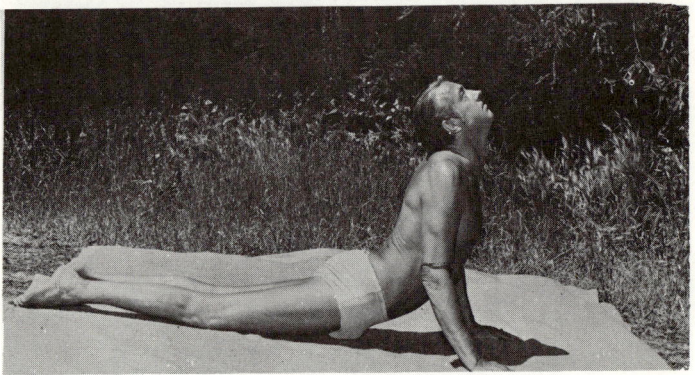

Cobra Pose (*Bhujangasana*)

After resting, following the Shoulder Stand, turn over on the stomach and place the hands on the floor beside the pectoral muscles. Arch upward, using the back muscles and pushing down to assist with the arms as necessary to complete the pose. Obtain as complete a stretching of the body as possible. Hold without straining and resume the starting position. Rest, then repeat three to five times. You will note that this pose complements the Shoulder Stand and provides stretch to the spine in the opposite direction. Muscles of the back, abdomen and entire upper body are strengthened by the practice of the Cobra Pose.

Asanas for Health and Mastery

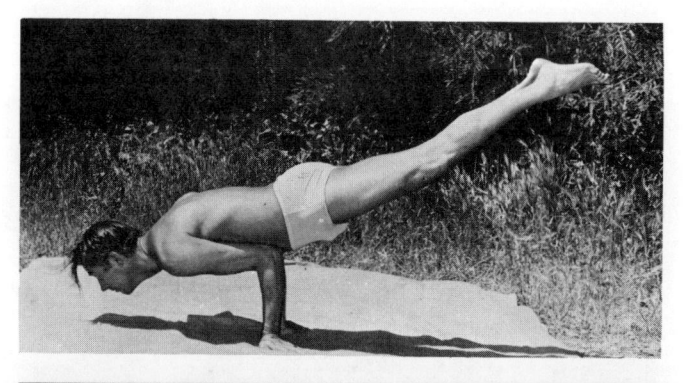

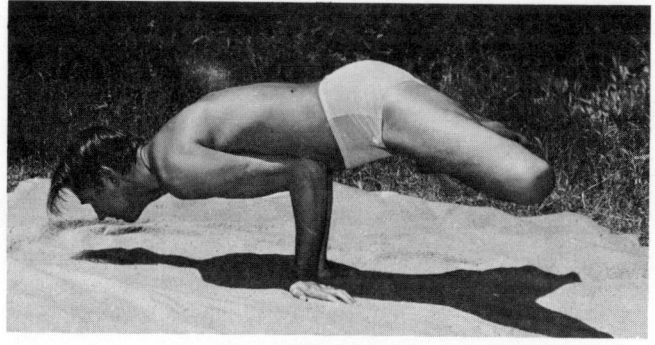

Peacock Pose (*Mayurasana*)

The Peacock Pose is not always easy for women to practice because of the placement of the upper arms. Since it is rather strenuous, some men will find that the modified pose is more comfortable, and the benefits are the same, without the strain sometimes felt in the completed pose. Assume the starting position, with elbows together and placed in the center of the abdomen. Lean forward, until balance is attained, and lift the feet from the floor. When needed, resume the beginning position and lie down to relax. Once or twice is enough for the average person to practice. The Peacock Pose strengthens the entire upper body and stimulates internal processes.

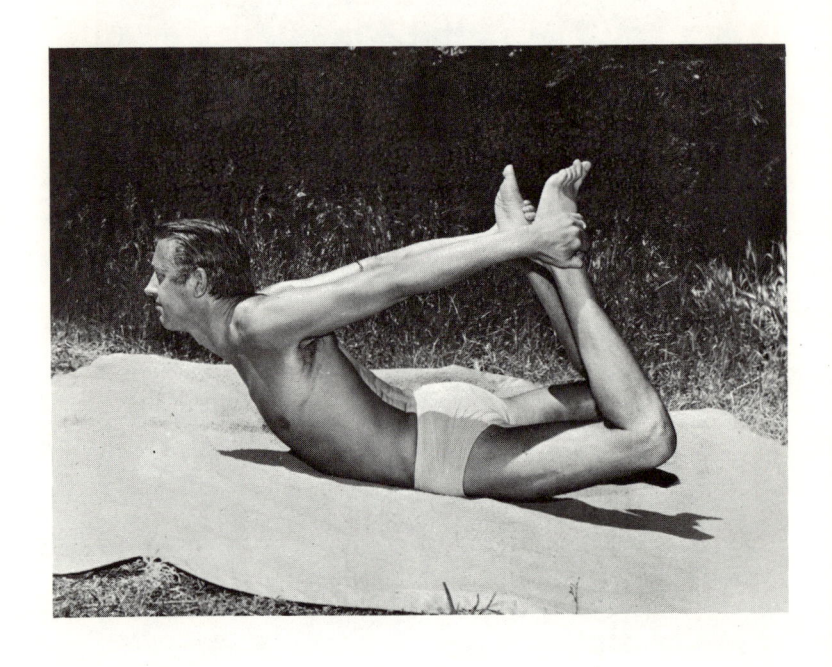

Bow Pose (*Dhanurasana*)

    Begin lying down on the stomach, reach back and grasp the ankles, then arching upwards, pull the body into the completed pose. Hold for as long as comfortable and relax. Repeat as inclined.

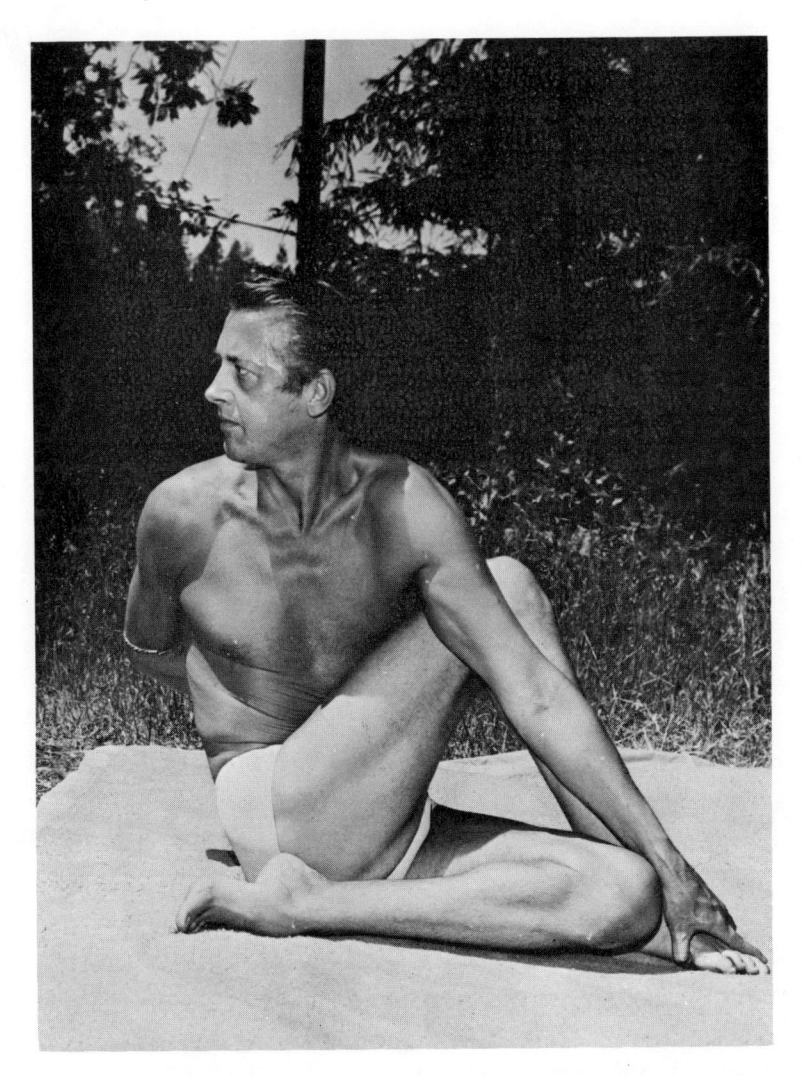

Half-Spinal Twist (*Ardha-Matsyendrasana*)

It is easier for one to follow the illustrations than to follow the written explanation. This pose increases flexibility of the body and imparts strength, while it effectively adjusts the spinal vertebrae.

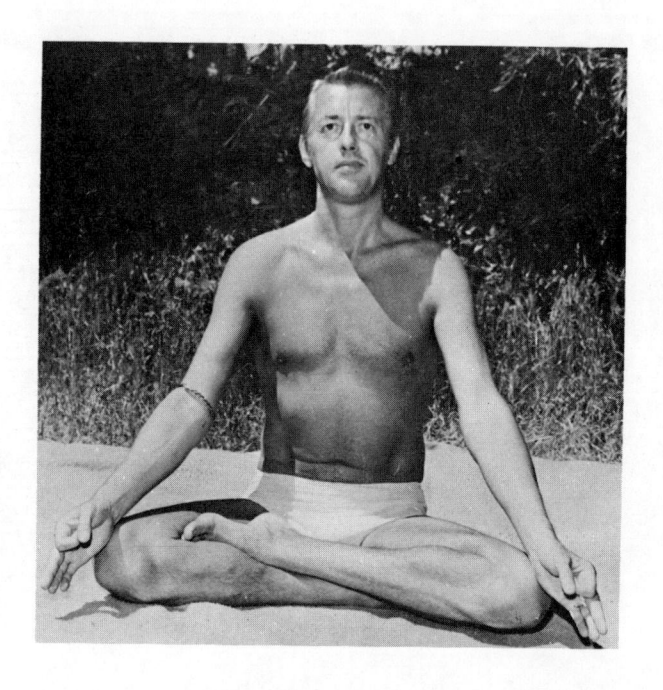

Perfect Pose (*Siddhasana*)

One of the most popular meditation postures is *Siddhasana*. The Sanskrit name means "Perfect Pose," because one attains perfection in Yoga by meditating in this position. *Siddhasana* is useful to learn, since it is used as the practice seat for some of the *pranayamas* and the *mudras*. The positions of the legs and the hands also contain the body energies by closing the circuits and allowing awakened vital forces to remain in the system during meditation practice. Place the heel of one foot at the juncture of the genitals and the anus. Arrange the other foot as nearly on top of the lower foot as possible. Sit up straight and arrange the hands on the knees. This is *Siddhasana*. Once this has been mastered, it is truly a comfortable position for meditation practice.

Asanas for Health and Mastery

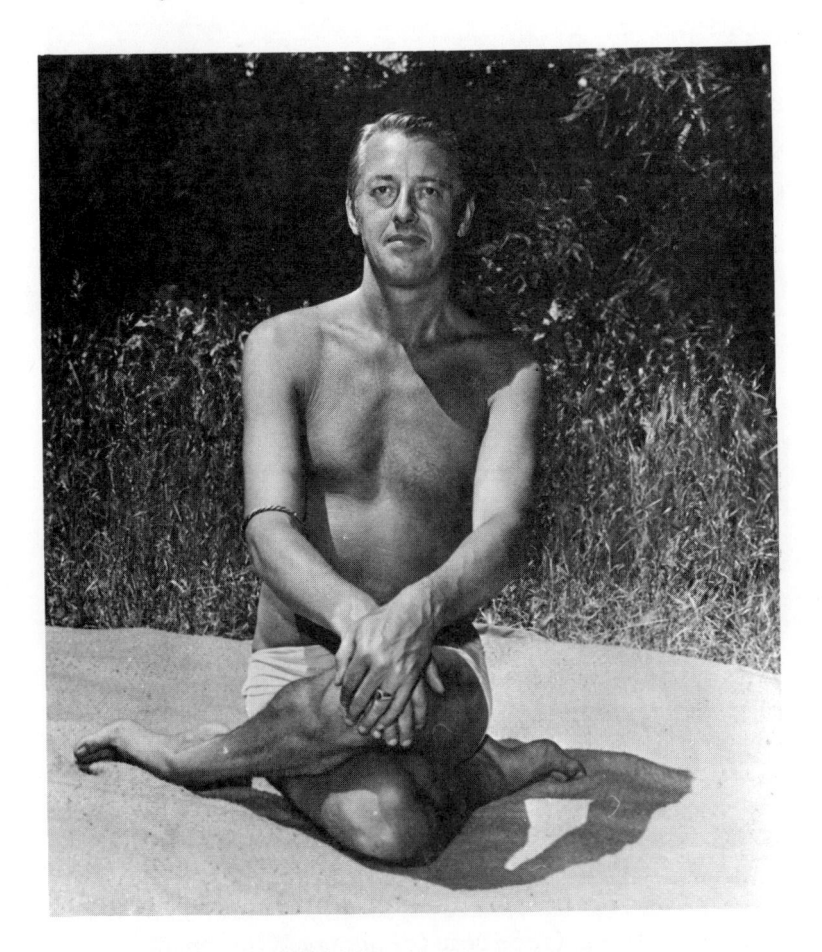

Dangerous Pose (*Samkatasana*)

The Dangerous Pose is another meditation position. The name is given, because the pose suggests one who is alert and in command. Variations in seated positions enable one to avoid inconvenience and fatigue, as well as to experience the distribution of energy flows encouraged by the placement of limbs and feet. This pose can be used for *mantra* practice or whenever a seated pose is required.

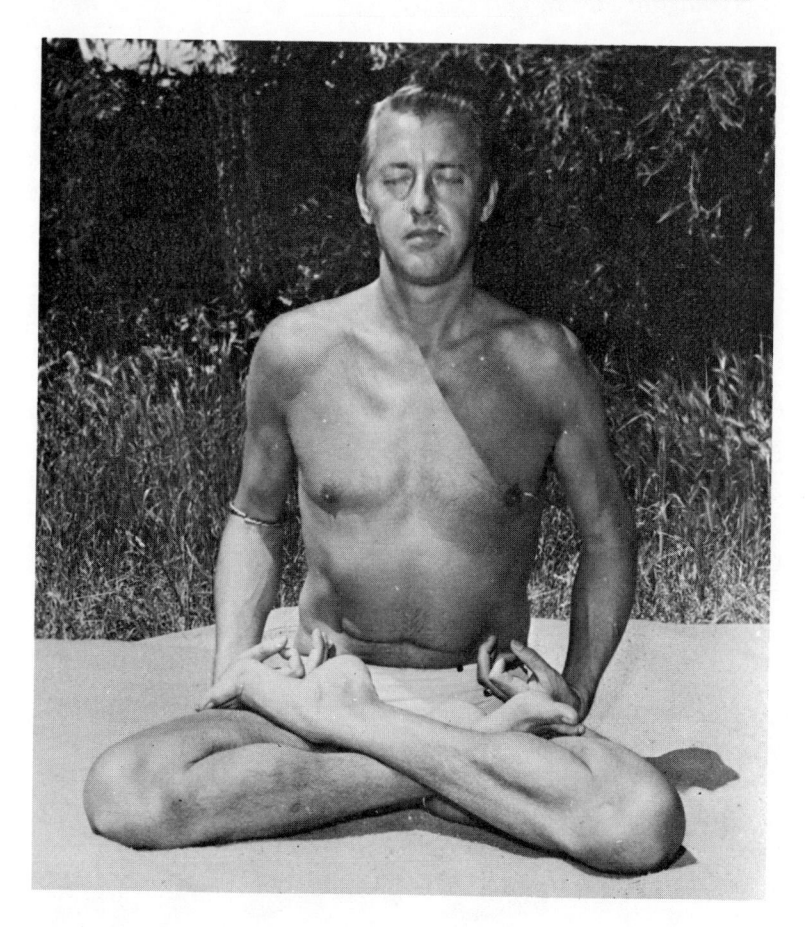

Lotus Pose (*Padmasana*)

    The yogi remains firm and stable in the Lotus Pose, while contemplating the *chakra* (lotus) centers within during meditation. This is a classic meditation position but is not always easy for westerners to master. It may take time for the ligaments to become extended so that the Lotus Pose is comfortable. If one cannot master the Lotus Pose, any of the other seated poses will do quite well for the purpose of meditation. Start slowly and acquire proficiency over a period of time.

Headstand (*Sirsasana*)

When learning the Headstand, it is a good idea to have a friend stand by to catch you, in the event of overbalancing, or to do it against a wall. Be sure to remain clear of furniture, windows and any condition which might prove dangerous should balance be lost. Gradual practice will bring results. Placement of the hands can be as shown, with the three-pointed position being easier for most persons in the beginning. Hold the position as long as comfortable without strain. Usually a few seconds will suffice to begin with, longer when ease of the posture is experienced. When coming down from the pose, do so in a controlled manner and remain face down, as shown, for a few moments, until the blood circulation has normalized in order to avoid dizziness.

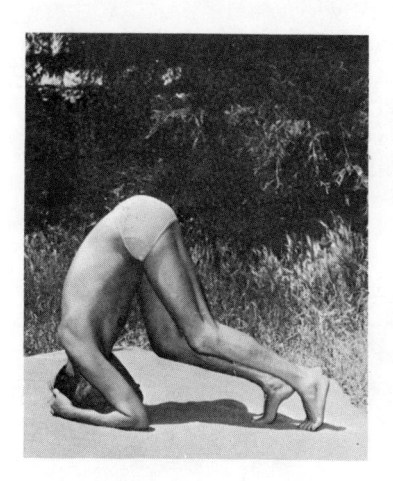

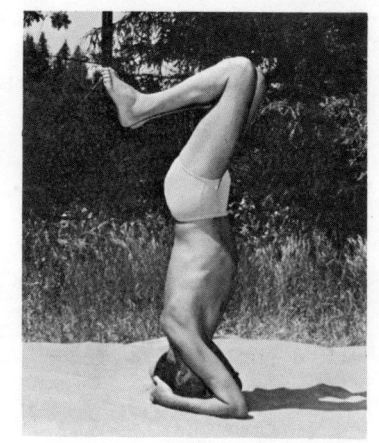

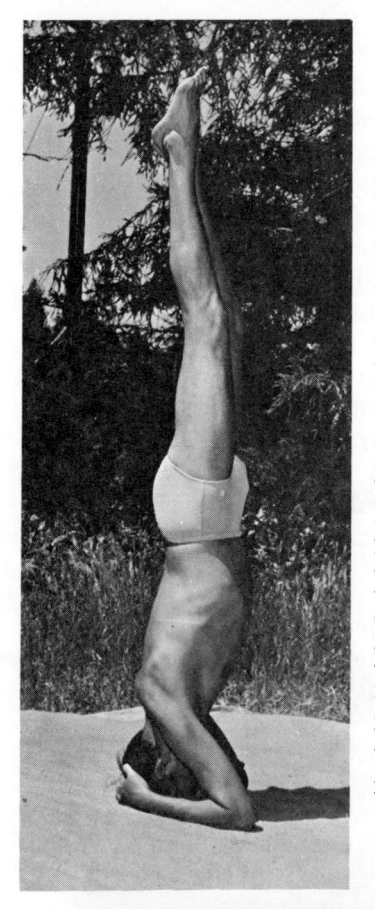

Resting in this manner takes pressure off lower limbs, rests the heart and sends a rich supply of blood to the brain. The Headstand should not be practiced by persons who are overweight, have heart trouble, high blood pressure, problems with the bones in the neck or cataracts in the eyes. The endocrine glands are powerfully influenced by the practice of the Headstand, which is why it is so highly extolled by teachers of yoga as a great rejuvenator. Those who cannot practice the Headstand can derive benefit from the Shoulder Stand. If this is not possible, then the regular use of a slant board is recommended.

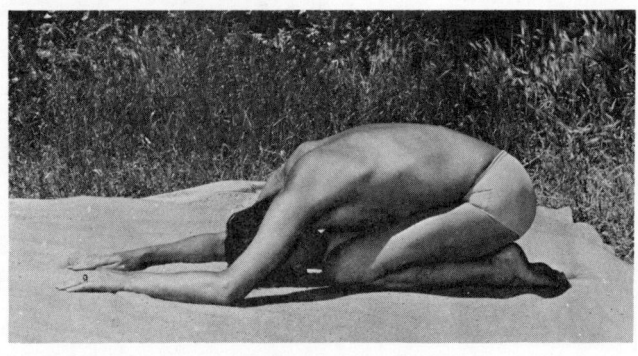

Experience in the practice of *Yogasanas* will confirm their contribution to health and a sense of well-being. For the body to function normally, there must be sufficient blood circulation to carry nutrients throughout the system, to provide oxygen and to carry off carbon dioxide and other wastes. The lymphatic system must function normally, and the glands must do their work. It is obvious that flexibility of the spine is encouraged by the practice of most asanas. For persons in need of spinal correction, it will be advisable to obtain the services of a chiropractic physician, who will make the necessary manual adjustments to insure that nerves are not impinged and that the currents flowing through the system are not impeded.

Yogasanas are best practiced on an empty stomach, with a short rest taken afterward (either in the Corpse Pose or during meditation in the seated position which is most comfortable), so that the effects can be retained by the body.

If one is going from *asana* practice, into the *pranayamas* and *mudras* and on to meditation, the complete program can be accomplished in one session.

Chapter Five
PRANAYAMAS FOR REGULATING VITAL FORCES

Pranayama means the regulation or control of vital force in the system. The easiest way to control the circulation of vital force is through regulating the process of breathing, because there is an interrelationship between the circulation of air in the nasal passages and lungs and the movements of vital force in the system. These methods are, therefore, the most direct route to control of *prana*.

Pranayama purifies the blood, brain, nerves and subtle tissues of the body. When the body becomes luminous through the practice of *prayanama*, one is said to shine like a god.

If one is to include the regular practice of *pranayama* as part of a daily routine, the following beginning exercise is recommended. Sit in a meditation pose and be relaxed. Close the eyes and feel the *prana* in the spinal pathway. Inhale and hold the breath, mentally chant the mantra *lam* in gentle rhythm, while feeling the location of the base *chakra*. Exhale when the need is felt. Do not strain. Resume normal breathing until comfortable. Then, move up to the sacral *chakra*, inhale, hold, and repeat the mantra *vam* for the duration of breath retention. Relax. Go on doing this with each *chakra* in order: *ram* mantra at the solar plexus; *yam* mantra at the heart *chakra*; *ham* mantra at the throat *chakra*. Then, relax and prepare for the *pranayamas* to follow.

At any time when the fire element of the body needs to be stimulated, hold the left nostril closed and breathe for a while through the right nostril. If the body is too hot and coolness is needed, breathe for a while through the left nostril. Air moving through the right

Pranayamas

nostril encourages a greater volume of current to flow through the right channel (*pingala*), and air flowing through the left nostril causes a greater volume of current to flow through the left channel (*ida*); these are the sun and moon currents, respectively. When these currents are even in force of flow, the *kundalini* tends to awaken and ascend upward through the central pathway (*sushumna*), making meditation easier and even spontaneous.

Ujjayi Pranayama is a prerequisite to some of the *kriya* practices and has a beneficial influence upon the entire nervous system. Open the throat by relaxing it, keeping the mouth closed. Inhale through the nostrils, making a mild sound as the air is inhaled, hold. Repeat a half dozen times or more.

Sheetali Kumbhak tends to quench thirst and hunger and calms body and mind. It also cools the system. Open the mouth a little, roll the tongue into a tube (or try to) and inhale through the mouth, hold. Ten to fifteen times is usually adequate.

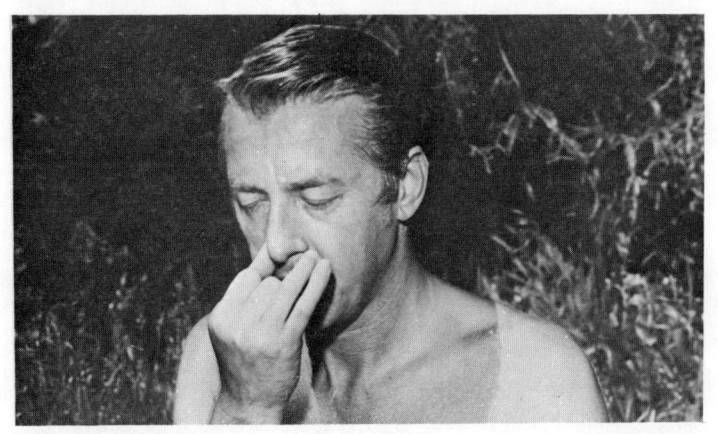

Alternate Nostril Breathing is one of the most commonly practiced *pranayamas*. I know of one man who was advised by his guru to practice this for twenty minutes each morning without fail. He told me that whenever he did it, he perspired before his session was over. Ordinarily, we recommend that one practice ten cycles to begin with, then increase slowly, always remaining within range of personal comfort and capacity. The process is simple. Just arrange the thumb and fingers at the nostrils, inhale through the left nostril . . . hold for as long as comfortable . . . exhale through the right nostril . . . hold for as long as comfortable . . . inhale through the right . . . hold, exhale through the left. Repeat. This is a powerful yet easy *pranayama* to be practiced on a regular basis, as it will cleanse the *nadis* and balance the flow of vital forces.

Bhastrika means "bellows," and it is easy to see why this *pranayama* is so named. Exhale completely, let the air into the lungs naturally (it will flow back into the lungs once the air has been vigorously expelled) and continue the vigorous expulsion and inhalation with a rapid bellows action. Let the air come into the nose at the tip of the nose. Ten, twenty or even thirty such expulsions and inhalations can take place in sequence. Inhale, exhale and rest. Repeat without becoming tired. This practice pushes stale air out of the lungs and awakens vital forces throughout the system.

The preceding *pranayamas* are those most commonly taught and used. There are many others which are taught, including variations of all of them, according to the inclination of the *guru*. Some teachers stress only a few *pranayamas*, and others run their disciples through all of them. My view is that one who is intent on the yogic path should become proficient in all techniques, in order to be able to speak from experience when instructing students as well as to gain the benefits of practice. There is a connection, obviously, between mind and body (between the non-material and the material). These basic exercises afford one the opportunity of learning just how this connection is made, as well as how to encourage health, function and ultimate realization of Supreme Consciousness. Yogis teach that conscious breathlessness is deathlessness. Ordinarily, when the involuntary nervous system is exhausted, we go to sleep for a few hours. When complete exhaustion is experienced, we make our transition. With *Raja Yoga* meditation, a yogi can rest the involuntary nerves consciously and extend his stay in the body to work out *karma*, to perform useful service and to complete his quest for liberation of consciousness.

An advanced yogi knows and prepares for the time of his transition by making sure no subtle earth attachments remain and by consciously meditating at the hour of transition to detach his consciousness from the body, mind and feeling nature. In this manner, he performs *mahasamadhi*, the "great samadhi," and transcends lower worlds in favor of higher ones; he even awakens to the clear state with no attachment or identification with matter at all.

The *Siddha Yoga* tradition to which I belong teaches that the body can be purified through the practice of Yoga so that the light of the soul shines through it with no obstructions. This is why even advanced yogis of this tradition attend to the regular practice of *yogic kriyas*, either intentionally performed or allowed to manifest spontaneously. The *kriyas* or cleansing actions work on a subtle level to transform the body and the nervous system astrally. It is true that a person who lives in an ideal environment, with pure air, good food, peace of mind, and who experiences *yogic kriyas*, can refine the body and mental field in one incarnation and experience liberation of consciousness. The traditional teaching is that, according to past *karma* and present effort and involvement, the purification process takes three years, six years, twelve years, twenty-four or forty-eight years. These cycles are not fixed, because some begin their work with much to cleanse from the system, while others come into the world with very little to work out.

Even with the practice of *pranayama* and *yogic kriyas*, one should meditate, contemplate and use powers of discrimination to discern that which is Real, in contrast to that which is subject to change.

Chapter Six
MUDRAS: AWAKENING KUNDALINI AND ACQUIRING CONSCIOUS CONTROL OVER THE INVOLUNTARY NERVOUS SYSTEM

Special exercises were discovered by yogis that would contribute to the awakening of *kundalini shakti* and allow this force to move freely through the *nadis* or channels throughout the body. Because of the circulation of the energy and because of conscious attention to the practice of these exercises, the current is made to flow upward through *sushumna* to the brain centers. One is also able to acquire conscious control over the systems of the body which are, in most persons, involuntary.

These exercises are called *mudras*. A *mudra*, in yogic practice, is a combination pose (*asana*) and technique for the control and regulation of life-force (*pranayama*) and is believed by some to be superior to either *asana* or *pranayama* alone. With *asanas*, one is primarily concerned with preparing the body for higher Yogas. With *pranayama* one gains control over the vital forces in the system and effectively practices withdrawal of the senses. With *mudras* one awakens *kundalini* and attains final mastery over body, vital forces and mental activity, and he is also able to allow a condition in which *samadhi* is naturally and easily experienced.

There are various yogic traditions, some stressing attention to *mudra* practice and others not. It is only a matter of teaching tradition, for one tends to teach what he has found useful for himself. There should be no attempt on the part of a *guru* to discredit the traditions of other qualified and authentic *gurus*. The texts stress that *mudras* should be practiced after having been taught by a *guru* who has, himself, mastered the exercises and gained the benefits. Such a *guru* is not only sure to teach correctly but also sure to be able to guide the disciple along the path so that awakening and unfoldment is natural and safe.

Two approaches are popular in regard to *mudra* practice: the first emphasizes the idea of purposeful practice of *mudras* to prepare the nervous system for awakened *kundalini* and to become consciously acquainted with the processes that take place; the second suggests that *kundalini* awakening through contact with the *guru* is of primary importance, with the *mudras* then taking place automatically. It would seem that both views are valid, for if the student actually learns *mudra* practice from the *guru*, he also will be attuned to the *guru's* consciousness so that *Shaktipat* will occur when conditions are ripe for it. What is suggested is that one should not try to practice *mudras* without the guidance of the *guru* or hope that *kundalini* awakening will result in *samadhi* states without the company of the *guru* or his useful counsel. In brief, one would not practice *mudras* without the *guru's* instruction, and there would be no danger of the disciple making a mistake.

It has been observed that when *shakti* becomes active, many of the *mudras* are practiced spontaneously without the disciple ever having been taught how to do them. *Mudras* were probably developed both from observing spontaneous happenings during yogic *kriyas*, which took place when *shakti* became active, and by experimentation to encourage *shakti* activity and to gain control over the involuntary systems.

If the disciple has observed the rules and regulations, which are the prerequisite of yogic practice, and is instructed by the *guru* to practice *mudras*, then all will be in order. If the preliminary requirements have not been met and if the *guru* has not given instruction, then one should not practice *mudras*. To try to practice *mudras* without preparation and without personal instruction would be an irresponsible act. One who is not responsible is not likely to attain any degree of success on the yogic path.

There are several *mudras* described in various yogic texts which are said to give *siddhi* (perfection) to the practitioner. These practices are to be kept secret by the yogi for two reasons: (1) if one wastes energy and time discussing personal practices with others, energy is drained from the system that could better be used in practice; (2) the instruction of the *guru* to the disciple is for the disciple's welfare alone—to pass on information received from the *guru*, after one has been pledged to secrecy, is both a breach of faith and unfair to the other person, if he has not been prepared for instruction in the correct manner. Yogic *kriyas* should only be taught to persons who have prepared themselves as a result of the practice of preliminary techniques and procedures. A few of the *mudras* will now be explained.

Mahamudra (Great Mudra)

Sitting on the floor, place the left heel at the juncture of the anus and the genitals. Extend the right leg. Draw the current up the spine by contracting the sphincters of the anus and sucking the current up with *kriya* breath. Hold the breath, keep the attention at the third eye and bend forward to grasp the foot. Hold for a moment, stretch the spine. Sit upright and relax as the current descends. Reverse leg positions and repeat the process. Then, extend both legs and repeat. This is *Mahamudra*.

In the beginning, it can be practiced six to twelve times. Advanced yogis do it as many as one-hundred and forty times. This *mudra* will stir *kundalini* into action and direct the energy upward through the system.

Sky Mudra (Nabho Mudra)

The Sky Mudra is a useful practice when resting between *mudra* practices. Sit in a comfortable meditation

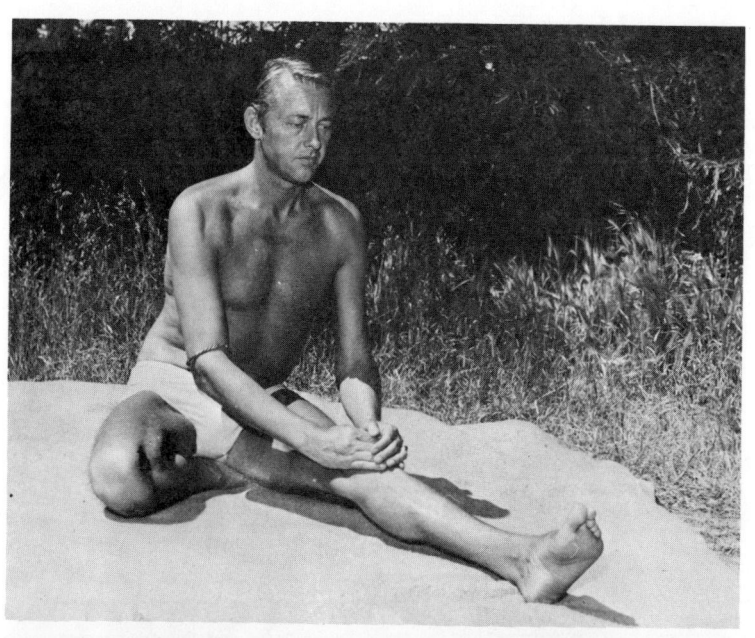

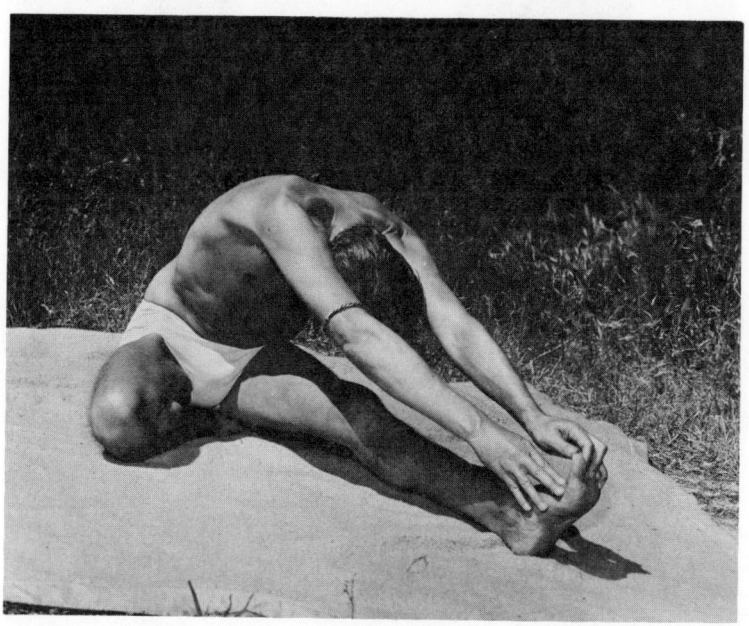

pose with attention flowing to the third eye. Roll the tongue back into the throat cavity, as nearly as possible, and press upward against the back part of the mouth. Hold this position for a while. This results in subsidiary salivary glands being forced to secrete fluids, which can then be swallowed. This process provides useful substances to the body and encourages body function and improved health.

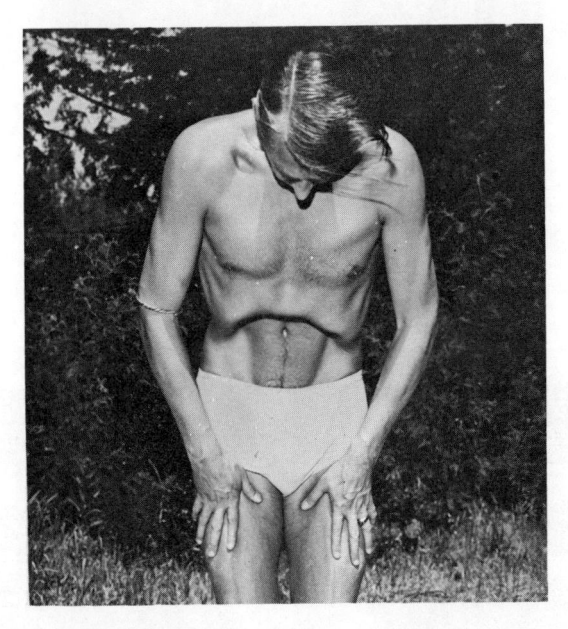

Stomach Lift (Uddiyana Bandha)

Uddiyana means to "fly up," and this *mudra* allows one to draw the abdominal muscles up into the chest cavity. At least this is how it appears when practiced. This practice increases digestive fire, beneficially influences the adrenal glands, brings great energy to the solar plexus and massages the internal organs. It is very useful in awakening *kundalini*. *Uddiyana* is easily learned, simple to practice and the benefits are many.

Stand and lean over, placing the hands on the thighs

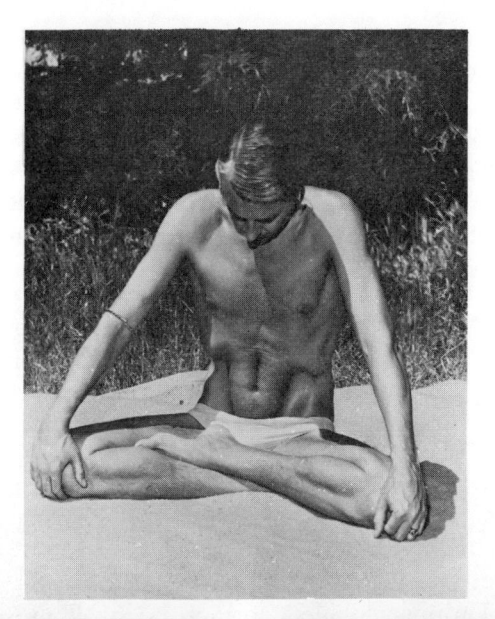

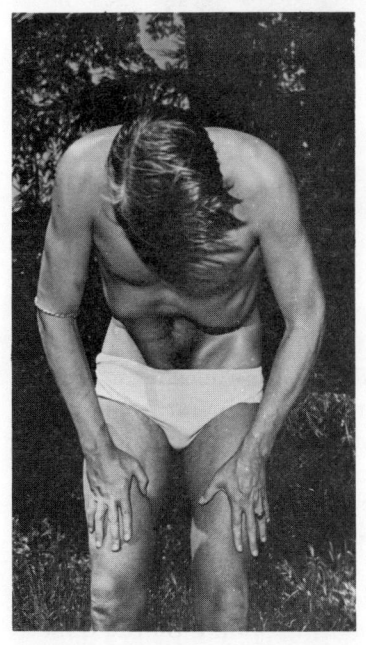

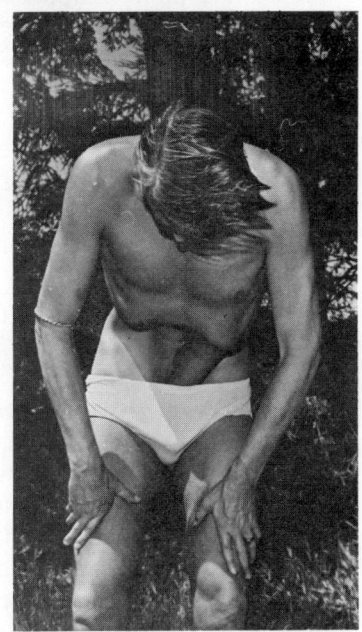

Mudras: Awakening Kundalini

without exerting any downward pressure. Inhale, then exhale and keep the lungs empty. Lift the chest cavity and suck in; the result will be that the stomach area is drawn up and back. The key here is to keep the abdominal muscles relaxed. The effect is realized by the inward sucking area. Suck up and in, hold, release and relax. With practice one can perform a number of rapid "lifts" on one breath—as many as twenty or thirty or more. Start with a few rounds to avoid becoming tired. Then, as capacity increases, do more. Advanced procedure would be to do twenty or thirty on a single breath and then rest a few moments. Then, do another set. Then, another. Three sets of several "lifts" are adequate.

Throat Lock (Jalandhar Bandha)

This *mudra* beneficially influences the thyroid gland and gives control of breath and vital force. Sitting in a meditation pose, inhale, contract the throat muscles and press the chin against the upper part of the chest. Let the attention flow to the third eye. Hold for as long as comfortable, then inhale. Breathe normally a few times and repeat.

Anal Contraction (Mulbandha)

Sit in *Siddhasana* with the left heel under the anus and the right foot over the genitals. Contract the muscles of the anus and genitals, pulling up and in with muscular effort and with the abdominal muscles. Hold for as long as comfortable. Relax. Repeat a few times. This will give conscious control over the nerves and the muscles of the organs of elimination and generation and will stir energies in the lower *chakra*. When the energies are awakened, they can then be raised upward through *sushumna* in meditation. One should also perform the throat lock when practicing this *mudra*. In sequence: inhale; perform the throat lock; contract and lift the muscles of anus, genitals and abdomen; hold and relax;

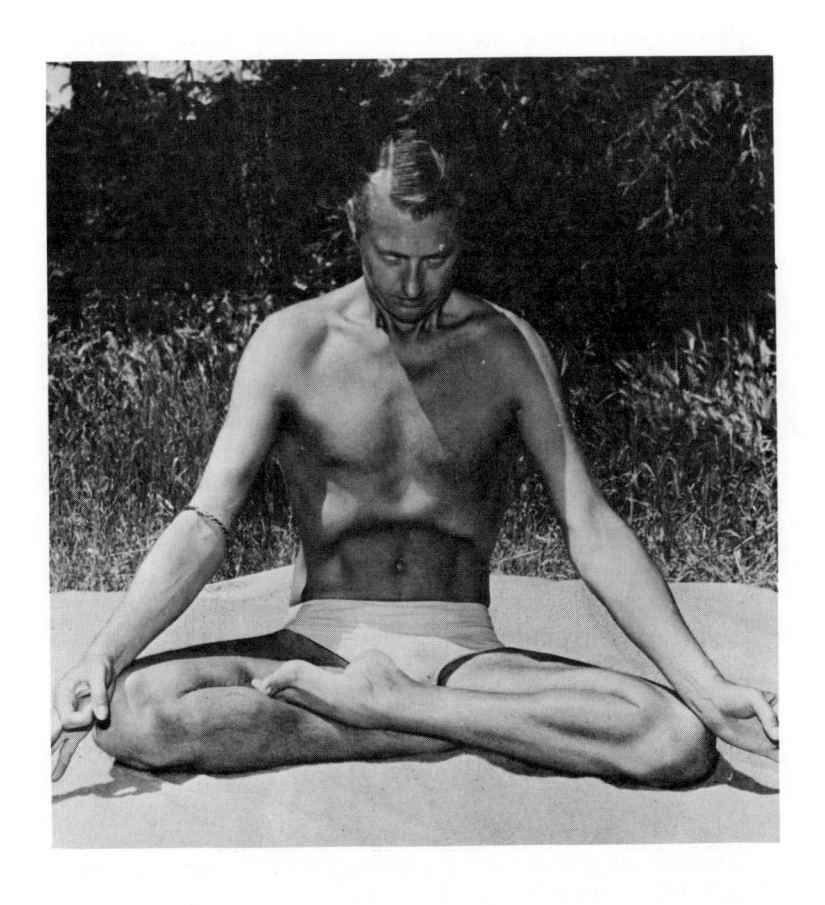

repeat. When done in this manner it is also called *Mahabandha*, or "Great Lock," because it prevents the downward flow of energy by closing off possible openings.

(Khechari Mudra)

Very rarely practiced, even among avid Yoga students, is this unique exercise. In the *Sky Mudra*, we rolled the tongue back toward the throat cavity and pressed upward against the top of the mouth to encourage secretions of the salivary glands. In *Khechari Mudra*, one is taught how to massage and stretch the tongue daily in order to be able eventually to roll it back and insert it behind the palate into the nasal cavity. Yogic texts assert that certain nerves are located in this cavity, which are stimulated by the placement of the tongue. Also, one who is practicing prolonged *samadhi* states will be so relaxed that breathing becomes minimal, even stopping for a length of time. The placement of the tongue in the cavity behind the palate helps to keep *shakti* concentrated in the higher brain centers and steadies it there. This happens automatically in some instances, when *kundalini* becomes active and flows strongly upward into the crown *chakra*. Not all yogis who experience the superconscious states experience *Khechari Mudra*, and there are many enlightened persons who know nothing about it. This practice is not essential to the enlightenment experience. It is simply one of the techniques which have been used by yogis to acquire control of body energies and functions.

(Vipreetkari Mudra)

This mudra is a rejuvenation exercise, to be sure. The practice is simple. It is the same as the Shoulder Stand (*Sarvangasana*). Assume the position and hold for as long as comfortable. This beneficially influences the thyroid, pituitary and adrenal glands. It sends a rich blood supply to the head and gives rest to the lower

Mudras: Awakening Kundalini

extremities. The esoteric teaching, relative to this practice, is that it prevents the downflow of energies from the brain and allows them to be absorbed there, instead of being spent in lower body functions.

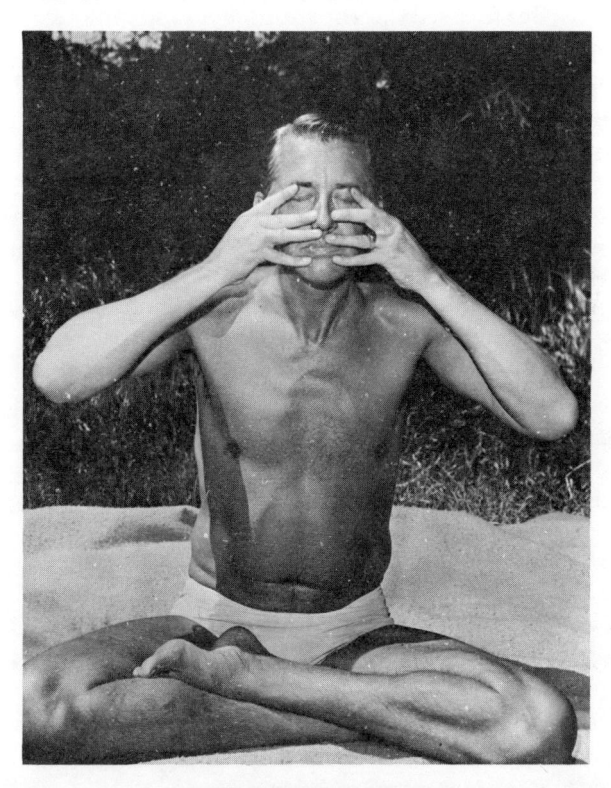

(Yoni Mudra)

This is one of the most useful exercises to practice, because it allows concentration and meditation on the *chakra* system and gives control over the vital forces in the body. Sit in *Siddhasana* or any comfortable position. Close the ears, eyes, nostrils and mouth as shown in the illustration. There are variations in the practice of this *mudra*, and the approach can change from one meditation session to another.

a. Draw the current up with the *kriya* breath to the third eye center. Be centered here, looking within and listening within to the internal sound. Merge in the light and sound.

b. Be focused at the third eye and practice with *mantra* such as *Ham-Sa* or *So-Ham* (Ham sounds like "Hum"). In time, flow into the crown *chakra* and beyond it. Rest here.

c. Draw the current up, one *chakra* at a time, and concentrate for a while at each *chakra*, trying to see the inner light reflected from each one and hearing the inner sound emanating from each one; continue gradually until reaching the crown *chakra*, resting here.

d. Contemplate the ideal, "Supreme Consciousness am I," while absorbed in the crown *chakra*.

The practice of this *mudra* is a useful method for the experience of *samadhi*. Closing the ears, eyes, nose and mouth, one is totally inwardly directed.

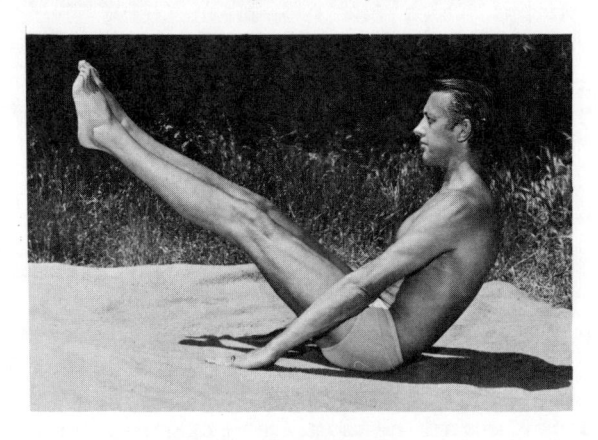

(Vajroni Mudra)

Sit on the floor with legs extended. Place palms on the floor and raise the body. This strengthens the body and imparts vitality. This *mudra* causes vital forces to flow upward. Sex energies are converted into subtle force with the practice of this *mudra*.

(Shambhavi Mudra)

Sit in a meditation pose and direct the eyes towards the middle of the eyebrows, the third eye center, and contemplate your true nature as Supreme Consciousness. This practice controls breath, *prana* and thought processes. Inner vision is opened by this practice, and one is able to move through the door to higher realms. The third eye is the connecting point between the higher and the lower realms. It is through this astral doorway that one can enter the subtle realms at will and see what transpires there. One can practice this *mudra* while practicing *Yoni Mudra*, look into the third eye to see the lights of the lower *chakras* reflected there, hear their sounds and understand the nature of the five elements regulated by the *chakras*. Contemplating the five *chakras* and understanding the nature of the elements, one is said to be performing the *five contemplation mudras* which give supreme mastery. There are *mantras* to be inwardly recited at each *chakra*; *lam* at the base *chakra*, *vam* at the sacral *chakra*, *ram* at the lumbar *chakra*, *yam* at the heart *chakra*, *ham* at the throat *chakra*, *ksham* at the third eye, and *bam* at the crown *chakra*. These *mantras* quicken the energies and cause them to ascend. They are pronounced with a long sound to the *a*, as in "law." One can experiment by chanting these *mantras* aloud and feeling the response in the respective *chakras*.

1. *Earth Element Contemplation*—After making a study of the earth element, one looks into the third eye, while feeling the base *chakra* and contemplating the nature of the earth element. One can chant the *mantra* *lam* and feel the energies stir, before settling down to contemplation.

2. *Water Element Contemplation*—Look into the third eye while feeling the sacral *chakra* and contemplate the water element. One can chant the *mantra* *vam* and feel the energies stir at the beginning of this contemplation.

3. *Fire Element Contemplation*—Look into the third eye, and feel and retain *prana* in the lumbar *chakra* and solar plexus. Chant the *mantra ram* to start. Then contemplate the meaning of the fire element.

4. *Air Element Contemplation*—Look into the third eye and retain *prana* at the heart *chakra*. Chant the *mantra yam* to start. Then contemplate the air element.

5. *Ether Element Contemplation*—Look into the third eye and hold the *prana* steady at the throat *chakra*. Chant the *mantra ham* to begin the practice. Contemplate the nature of the ether element.

Yogic texts claim that *siddhis*, occult powers, are obtained by successful practice of these techniques. Mastery over the earth element gives one power over the body to remain forever youthful; mastery over water enables one to avoid accidents involving water; mastery over the fire element enables one to avoid accidents with fire; mastery over the air element slows the process of metabolism and gives power to move through space (in consciousness); mastery over the ether element makes one independent of gross food and gives access to subtle spaces. Literally, one overcomes the world as a result of these practices.

Chapter Seven
YOGIC INITIATION AND MEDITATION TECHNIQUES

Some benefit is, of course, derived from the practice of yogic methods, even if one is not personally initiated by a *guru*. There are at least two reasons why personal initiation is advised: one, the disciple is assured of receiving an authentic method, clearly explained and correctly advised; two, at initiation, if conditions are ideal, the disciple receives from the *guru* an infusion of current, which awakens the disciple's latent forces and starts them circulating.

Initiation can be given in simple circumstances or with an elaborate ceremony, depending upon the will of the *guru* and the need of the moment. What transpires between *guru* and disciple is to be kept secret and inviolate, because the instruction is for the disciple alone. Others can prepare themselves for their own initiation according to their need and receptivity.

Unfortunately, some high-powered organizations make use of the media to promise fantastic results to seekers who will come into their particular meditation system. There is nothing wrong with using the media as communication. What is contrary to yogic tradition is the big promise and the effort to recruit "disciples" en masse. To self-realized masters of Yoga, there are no "secret" or "special" systems; all of the basic techniques are known to these masters, who teach according to the need of the seeker.

There are inner schools and outer ones: esoteric and exoteric. There are methods prescribed for the masses, and there are methods given to the few who are ready to receive them. Even Jesus taught in parables (earthly stories with a heavenly meaning) for the people at large, but he taught the mysteries to the chosen few, who were ready for the truth stripped of all symbolism and myth.

Maharishi Mahesh Yogi is of the tradition of the Shankaracharyas and, therefore, is an initiate of Yoga who knows the complete system. He has chosen, as his mission, to inspire the masses to meditate; thus he gives a simple result-producing *mantra* method, which almost anyone can use with benefit. His work is of inestimable value. My line of *gurus* taught the total yogic way and privately geared the work to the needs and the capacities of those who were drawn. I work in this tradition. Swami Muktananda teaches *mantra* and the way to awakening through attunement with the *guru*. Then *kundalini* is aroused by this association and contact, and the *kriyas* take place spontaneously. All *Siddha* masters teach the same essential truth in basically the same manner, with the outer difference being a matter of tradition and personal style.

For centuries *Siddha gurus* have taught the way to purification and Enlightenment. Some give a few simple procedures; others stress the total program. Whatever the *guru* teaches is right for those who are drawn to him, according to karmic relationships and personal needs. There should be no argument between disciples of different traditions and no thought that one way is better than another. In this tradition, the *guru* teaches what he is destined to teach, and the disciple attracts to himself what he requires for his awakening and unfoldment.

Mantra is a basic meditation technique and is suitable for everyone. Even those whose destiny it is to go on to the more advanced *kriyas* practice *mantra* for purification, mind control and eventual absorption in OM. The primal sound (OM, Aum, Amen) is the sound of the current out of which everything comes into form. It is that into which everything eventually returns. It is the basic *mantra*, and all *mantras* dissolve into it. Specific *mantras* are used to awaken energies, to stimulate *chakras* and to clear the mind, as well as for other intended purposes. By understanding *mantra*, the science of sound, one can control the elements, cause or prevent rain, put out fires, heal the sick, awaken *shakti*, eradicate *karma*, produce solid objects by gathering together free energy in space, clear the mental field and achieve total mastery of the outer and the inner environment. Our concern here, however, is meditation and Self-Realization. Some common *mantras* follow.

So-Ham mantra is practiced while observing the natural flow of breathing. With inhalation, one mentally listens to the sound of "so," and, with exhalation, one listens to the sound of "ham" (hum), continuing until total relaxation ensues or the superconscious state is experienced. This is a potent *mantra*. It is natural and easy. Anyone can use it with benefit. It can be used for the duration of meditation or as a preliminary to the more advanced techniques in this *Siddha* Yoga tradition.

Ham-Sa mantra is used in the same manner. With *ham* (hum) one inhales and with *Sa* one exhales. Only the vibrational effect differs. Some texts inform us that this *mantra* becomes *So-Ham* as the body is relaxed and the mental state becomes more subtle; thus one could use *So-Ham mantra* from the beginning.

To deepen the practice, one might flow the attention to the third eye center and assume that air is flowing as current in through the third eye, down to the bottom of the spine with inhalation—and up and out through the third eye, as a flowing current, with exhalation. This will enable one to remain alert and attentive to the practice, instead of slipping into a borderline sleep state and repeating the *mantra* in a mechanical fashion.

Maha mantra is chanted aloud, while the preceding *mantras* are all done mentally. *Maha mantra* is also done quietly and then mentally. This *mantra* is designed to quicken the vital forces, bring energy up and inspire devotion. It is very effective. All of the words used are possessed of *mantra* power: *Hari Rama, Hari Rama,*

Rama, Rama, Hari, Hari . . . Hari Krishna, Hari Krishna, Krishna, Krishna, Hari, Hari. This is chanted with devotion for as long as one cares to chant it. The *Ram mantra* is especially effective in quickening the solar plexus *chakra* which, when strengthened, draws *kundalini* upward. Both Rama and Krishna were Indian *avatars*, but these names are *mantras*, as is the word *Christ*, which stirs the inner forces when heard or spoken.

For devotees of *Shiva* (the Holy Spirit aspect of the Godhead), there is a special *mantra*. It is chanted aloud to various musical scales or intoned mentally in harmony with the breathing cycle. If done in the inward way, it is mentally chanted with both inhalation and exhalation. With inhalation, one mentally chants *OM Namah Shivaya*; with exhalation, one chants *OM Namah Shivaya*, all the time contemplating the Reality of the Holy Spirit as Intelligence-Energy pervading the cosmos. It sounds like: *Om Namah Shivaya*. Once it is heard chanted, it is easy to duplicate.

One would not, of course, use all of the available *mantras* during one meditation session. It is best to remain with one *mantra* formula for several months in order to derive the benefits. It does not matter that we do not always relate to the meaning of the words of the *mantras*, for their effectiveness is in the influence of sound upon the body and the mind. If we do not know the meaning or if there is no meaning, these *mantras* are "seedless," in that we have no mental image in relationship to them. If we do have a mental image in relationship to a *mantra*, then it is *mantra* "with seed," and the image can be envisioned while the *mantra* is intoned or listened to mentally. For instance, for a mantra "with seed" (*bija mantra*), we might use *OM guru*. We could either listen to this *mantra* in the mind while inhaling and exhaling, or we might listen to one syllable with inhalation and to the other while exhaling . . . all the while visualizing the *guru* (or chosen ideal of God) at the third eye.

Here is a *mantra* I use quite often: after settling

down in a meditation position, I turn the attention to the third eye; then I think of Supreme Consciousness for a while; I let the mind think of God; then of the aspects of God (the Trinity, Christ Consciousness, Creative Energy-as-the-universe); next I visualize Babaji, the first in my line of *gurus*, and mentally intone, "Om Babaji, Om Babaji, Om Babaji" . . . until I feel the attunement with him. This is done in turn with Lahiri Mahasaya, Sri Yukteswar and Yoganandaji. When I finish, I may do *So-Ham mantra* or any of the *kriya pranayamas* before deeper meditation. After the techniques, I relax and let the flow of *kundalini* direct meditation. The attitude then is surrender and allowing God's grace to be operative.

Ramana Maharishi recommended the classic *mantras* according to the receptivity of those who came to him. One he recommended that anyone can use is this: watch the breathing rhythm and with inhalation mentally know, "I am"—with exhalation mentally know "Pure Consciousness." This is an affirmation of the truth of our being and is, therefore, a useful *mantra* to be contemplated and realized.

Those of a Christian background who reject Sanskrit *mantras* (because they are not comfortable with them) can use "OM Christ" or any useful combination of words as a *mantra*. The ideal with a *mantra* is to use it as a point of focus to direct attention, to flow with it and finally to transcend it.

A basic *mantra* is OM. It can be used on various levels: begin to audibly chant O-O-O-O-O-O-M-M-M-M-M-M-n-n-n starting low and ending with the sound in the top of the head. Feel it throughout the system. Chant it more quietly for a while. Whisper it for a while. Mentally chant it for a while. Listen to the mental sound for a while. Listen to the internal OM for a while. Transcend the *mantra*.

Some *mantras* easily get into the mental system and remain with us all the time. As they work, even when we are not consciously aware of them, they have a cleansing influence. When attention is released from the work at hand, the *mantra* floats to the surface of the mind, and we become aware of it. Since most people take in so much useless data in the course of the day, and their thoughts are random and wthout intention, it is well for one on the path to learn to use *mantra* correctly. As long as something is going on in the mind, at the conscious level as well as at the deeper levels, this "something" may as well be useful and constructive. *Mantra* and continual prayer is a way to purification of the sheaths of the soul and a way to liberation of consciousness.

The repetition of a *mantra*, usually a name of God, is called *Japa*. You may have seen a visiting Yoga teacher or a Tibetan lama fingering beads and moving the lips silently while walking, sitting or meditating. Beads are not necessary but are used as an aid to concentrating, as a reminder and to involve body movement (fingers) with mental chanting. The *mantra* can be a single word, a phrase, or whatever is useful and meaningful. *"Om Christ," "Om guru," "Om Namah Shivaya;"* any useful mantra will do. It is taught that the repetition of *mantra* for thousands of times strengthens the mind, purifies the body and results in the perfection of Yoga. Repetition of the *mantra* cleanses the subconscious of impressions and attracts the energies inherent in the *mantra* to one.

Sri Ram, Jai Ram, Jai, Jai, Ram OM is another powerful *mantra* that lends itself to group chanting, as well as to private audible or silent chanting.

Another popular *mantra* is *Govinda Jai Jai, Gopala Jai Jai, Radha Ramana Hari, Govinda Jai Jai.* Govinda and Gopala are names for Krishna in his various aspects. These *mantras* are best learned from someone who has been correctly taught by a *guru*, thereby utilizing the correct pronunciation and rhythm. Powerful devotion alone can make a *mantra* useful, by taking one's attention to the source of energy and thought, but, for the *mantra* effect, one should learn the correct intonation.

In the yogic tradition, *mantras* are usually given in Sanskrit for two reasons: first, the sounds used in this language are believed to have been received by (revealed to) sages during meditation; second, these sounds have been researched and tested for centuries, and their specific effects on the material environment are known. The sounds used in Sanskrit *mantras* carry with them the corresponding mental image or form. This is why they can cause effects in the physical environment if correctly utilized.

When the *guru* initiates his disciple, he does so according to need, time and circumstances. He may require elaborate preparation on the part of the disciple, or he may instruct the disciple and initiate him immediately, depending upon what is most useful for the disciple. If a disciple is receptive, he may be initiated immediately upon meeting the *guru*. Or, the *guru* may ask the disciple to practice yogic disciplines, purify the system mentally and physically and practice preliminary meditation methods for a time, in order to prove worthiness and to prepare for deeper work.

It is customary for the disciple to make a sacrifice (give something in return) for initiation. The real sacrifice is to burn the sense of ego in the flames of spiritual discipline and intense meditation. The outer ceremony usually requires that the disciple offer the *guru* a token of his life, in the form of money or substance which has been earned through work. Initiation cannot be purchased, but a flow of energy and evidence of open cooperation between disciple and *guru* must be visible. The *guru's* total life is given to awakening and liberating others; therefore, he wants to encourage the disciple to emulate him and become like him in understanding and in outlook on life. The offering given to the *guru* or the *guru's* cause is not payment for initiation; it is the disciple's way of sharing in the work and the ministry of the *guru* so that others can be served. By sharing his life, in the form of substance, the disciple shares his energy and consciousness with the *guru* and enters into a deeper relationship, which is spiritually beneficial.

One may seek instruction from one or several sources, as long as he is seeking the *way*. Once he is initiated by his *guru*, the search is over, and he can settle down to the practice of disciplines and methods which, over the years, will result in liberation of consciousness. Regardless of external teaching, the *way* to freedom in consciousness is from human consciousness to divine realization.

Chapter Eight
SUGGESTED ROUTINES OF PRACTICE

One who has been instructed in person by his *guru* will know the most useful routine for daily practice. It is well to learn all of the yogic methods in order to be informed, but for daily practice, the teachings of the guru should be followed to the letter. The attitude: "If one thing doesn't work, I'll try another," can lead to superficial practice and restlessness. Consider preliminary exercises as just that, preliminary. Devote the major portion of time and attention to the method stressed by your *guru*.

For a daily routine, this pattern might be followed: attend to cleansing of the body; practice *asanas, pranayamas* and *mudras*; meditate using the *mantra* or by flowing attention to the highest ideal; come out of meditation and begin the day with a cheerful attitude. The total session can take about an hour. On weekends, holidays and times of special retreat, more time can be given to meditation, both morning and evening.

Arrive at a schedule of practice which is useful and stick with it. If you drop out of meditation and want to continue, practice *mantra* or use any technique that will raise the *prana* and start the attention flowing back to the Transcendental Field.

During a prolonged meditation of one hour or more, whenever attention wanders, use a technique such as one of the *mudras* or any technique to regain concentration: contemplate the *chakras* one by one; flow into the third eye; flow into the crown *chakra*; listen to the internal sound; or simply let *kundalini* rise and carry you into deep meditation. When *kundalini* is very active, one will not have to work at meditation. Everything will occur naturally.

During occasions of retreat, when time is given fully to spiritual practices, a useful routine might be the following: in the morning, after cleansing, do the stomach exercises and some *pranayamas* (Alternate Nostril Breathing and the Bellows); meditate; have a glass of juice; go for a leisurely walk; read yogic texts or some inspirational material until mid-morning; practice *Yogasanas, pranayamas* and *mudras*; meditate deeply; rest a while, then have lunch; rest and study; practice *pranayama* and *meditate* in the early evening; rest and study; meditate before retiring for the night. In this way, one is fully involved with study, practice and periods of rest. During this time, avoid reading newspapers or listening to news reports. In fact, it is best during a retreat to disconnect the attention from worldly concerns entirely so that all energy and concentration can be directed to inner work.

Diet should be light but nutritious when we are engaged in intensive study and meditation. Much energy is expended in the practice of *mudras* and deep meditation, and fasting tends to weaken the body at such times. Balance and common sense is the rule at all times for one who would be successful on the yogic path. Too much sleep or too little is likewise to be avoided.

If strange visions occur or unsettling mental and emotional states become dominant, then relaxation and a cheerful attitude is recommended. There is nothing to fear on the yogic path, once we have been instructed by the *guru* and are open to inner guidance from the *guru* within us. If we are devoted on the path and surrendered to God, we will find that Innate Intelligence knows best what our experiences should be. We are God-led and God-sustained, always. Therefore, we should not fear. During occasions of confusion or temporary despair, read the *Bhagavad-Gita* and the lives of the saints. When I met my *guru*, he asked me to read only a few books the first year, as the major part of my time was to be given to practice of meditation and "living the life," so that I could have actual experience

Routines of Practice

instead of mere head knowledge. In addition to his books, I was to read the *Gita, The Practice of the Presence of God* by Brother Lawrence and *The Imitation of Christ* by Thomas A. Kempis. Later I was allowed to read more widely, once I had become attuned to my *guru's* consciousness and had become stable in meditation and discernment.

Being in a monastic environment, I practiced my disciplines and meditation in the morning and the evening and worked at least eight hours on the monastary grounds. On weekends and during retreats, I worked fewer hours and meditated up to eight hours a day, in two, three and five hour segments. With these long hours of meditation and a light vegetarian diet, I had a great deal of energy and slept four to five hours a night. Since *kundalini* was active and my *guru's* grace was operative, many unsought experiences were had: identification with the lights of the *chakras*; transcendental perceptions, astral visions, telepathic communication and dramatic inner changes.

During short or long retreats, it is helpful to be celibate so that all energy and thought can go into study and meditation. It is not uncommon for a person whose *kundalini* has started to awaken to feel strong sexual desire. This means that the energies are active in the lower *chakras*. When this energy is raised with the practice of *mantra* and yogic *kriyas*, it is used to refine and strengthen the higher centers. In the normal course of daily living, in a family situation, a natural sexual relation with one's mate will in no way interfere with success on the yogic path. The *Tantra* Yoga approach to sexual relations teaches that both parties should be fully in tune with one another and the sharing natural and spontaneous, with no ego motivation or strong need to make anything happen. The sexual relationship is then in harmony with nature and can actually contribute to expanded awareness and Cosmic Consciousness.

According to individual temperament, the practitioner of Yoga will organize his lifestyle. Simplicity is recommended and is in fact the natural outgrowth of dedicated yogic practice. Regardless of the scope of one's responsibilities, the personal life should be kept simple and well-ordered. A yogi can assume any lifestyle that Intelligence dictates, as long as he is true to himself and assuming the responsibilities which are his because of guidance, need for experience and *karmic* destiny. Masters of Yoga are very strict regarding this matter of responsibility to the world and to others. Yoga is not a path of escapism. This was the first thing Yoganandaji told me when I went to him for training. Some service must be rendered to the world in which we live. This can be in the form of service rendered to our fellowman, to our community and to nature. To take from the world without returning a useful contribution, according to our capacity and abilities, is to shirk our duty. *Living the life* is as important on the yogic path as is meditating and exploring the inner realms. If yogic practice results in our becoming small-minded, mean tempered, selfish, arrogant, proud of our accomplishments or self-serving, then we have missed the point. To those with greater understanding, more is expected, even demanded.

It is recommended that one have a special place for the practice of yogic disciplines. This can be a room which is used only for meditation and other routines. Two reasons are given for this: one, a personal space will assure us of privacy so that we can practice without interference; second, this practice area will become charged with *shakti* and contribute to uplift of energies when we practice. Also, memories of previous successful experiences in this place will awaken Consciousness and motivate one in a powerful way. An altar can be arranged nicely in this room, with photos of the *gurus* and saints and other objects which are meaningful to the yogi. Photographs inspire us and lift our attention to superconscious levels. There is a deeper significance, too, in that a photograph of a person acts as a point-of-contact with the one represented in the photograph and brings a stream of subtle energy from the person to the room through this visible object.

Prayer beads can be useful for intentional practice of *mantra*. *Rudraksha* beads are popular with yogis who feel attuned with the Holy Spirit (*Shiva*) aspect of the Godhead. They also have therapeutic influences on the body, since heat is conferred to the system by *rudraksha*—warming the heart and lungs when worn around the neck next to the skin and retaining *shakti* which is generated during meditation. Prayer beads can be of any material—wood, gemstone or a natural substance. Traditional with yogis of India are prayer beads (*japmala*) strung with one-hundred and eight beads, representing this many different names of God which are recognized and worshiped. For convenience, one-hundred beads to a string are useful and will enable one to keep count more accurately of *pranayamas* and *mantras*. A knot can be tied between the beads, or a larger bead can be used to mark the place (marking off ten, twenty, thirty or whatever number beads a person will require for ease in practice).

Assume, for the purpose of discipline, one decides to recite a prayer formula or *mantra* so many times a day, as discipline for controlling the mind and to avoid getting into a complacent rut during devotional practices. With the prayer beads rolled between the fingers, with each recitation one can give full attention to the inner work without having the distraction of also counting mentally. Any *mantra* will do: OM Guru, the *Maha Mantra* or whatever is preferred. In the practice of *pranayama*, if one has agreed within himself to do so many per sitting, the count can be done on the beads so that full attention can be given to practice and experience of *pranayama*.

Always, after intentional practice of techniques, sit in meditation with an attitude of surrender and let the meditation experience be spontaneous. Our intentional work is for the purpose of discipline, control of *prana*, awakening of *kundalini* and reversing the flow of attention from without to within. This is intentional, because we are doing it. After this intentional practice, we then flow our attention to the Source and become absorbed in It.

Here is a suggested routine that can either be adapted or modified to suit personal needs.

1. *Attend to morning cleansing.* Water used in bathing the body will balance electrical activity in the system.

2. Practice *asanas, pranayama* and *mudras.* If more time is given to this, do a complete routine. If less time is given, then do the stomach exercises (*Uddiyana Bandha* and *Nauli*) and the Shoulder Stand or the Headstand. Do Alternate Nostril Breathing and the Bellows breathing. Do *Maha Mudra.*

3. Sit for meditation. Pray, chant and invoke in your consciousness the reality of God's presence. Perform whatever preliminary techniques you have decided to do or those which have been prescribed by your *guru*: such as *Kriya Yoga, pranayama, Yoni Mudra* and *mantra.* Be absorbed in the awareness of Supreme Consciousness.

4. Come out of meditation with a feeling of joy and gratitude. Love and bless the world with your thoughts.

Chapter Nine
THE MESSAGE OF THE SIDDHAS

The perfect masters of Yoga are known as *Siddhas*, those who have attained perfection by recalling their divine nature and who work in harmony with the cosmos with total understanding. When liberation is attained in this incarnation, through diligent effort and the purifying activity of *kundalini*, one is referred to as *jivan-mukta*. *Jiva* is "soul" and *mukta* is the "condition of spiritual freedom." Beyond this is the stage where the body is transformed into a vehicle of light, where the person works through this body for the duration of his involvement with the universal cycles. One at this stage, with the transmuted body, is known as *para-mukta*, having gone beyond *maya* and the influence of nature. A *para-mukta* is supremely free and chooses, according to Divine will, to play a role in the world process. When a *Siddha* does any work at all, he knows: "Not I, but the Father (God) is doing the work." A *Siddha* master has no sense of ego and is not impelled by *karmic* compulsion. One who is in the *Siddha* tradition, who has not yet experienced total illumination and the transmuted body, will still have *karma* to work out and disciplines with which to be engaged.

Siddha masters usually teach according to a traditional pattern, but if they seem to work outside of tradition, they cannot be faulted, for they only do what is needful according to inner sanction. While usually working within the framework of natural laws, they can and sometimes do exercise their freedom to operate more subtle laws, which the average person does not comprehend. This is why it is taught that to be a disciple of a *Siddha* master is to be open to the flow of grace and Divine intervention. As we attune ourselves to the consciousness of a *Siddha* master, we partake, according to our own receptivity, of his realization and energy. Yoganandaji, in the *Siddha* tradition, would tell us, "Tune in with me and you will be attuned to God." Again, he would say, "I give you everything and hold nothing back. But you have to prepare yourself to receive what I have to give."

One may be faithful in the practice of yogic disciplines for decades and realize some benefit, for no sincere effort is ever wasted. But, when one is attuned to a *Siddha* master, one's spiritual progress is accelerated because of the grace of God flowing through such a master and because contact with him results in *shaktipat* (the transfer of his energy into our system which stirs *kundalini* into action). When *kundalini*, "the dormant potential energy," is awakened and begins to ascend to the crown *chakra* or *sahasrara*, the vital centers are activated, and the body-transmutation process is started. The descent of *prana* produced the physical form, the ascent transmutes the physical form.

Shaktipat takes place when the disciple is ready, for the teaching is that Innate Intelligence knows when to stir the force. The *guru's* presence can be the influence in our lives which awakens *kundalini*. Even if the *guru* is not physically present, through attunement with him and the line of *Siddha* masters he represents, the current can flow and contact can be made. I was quickened spiritually in my teenage years due to an active prayer life, to yearning for God-Realization and to the force of *samskaras*, which carried over from my previous life-cycle. But it was only after a few weeks with my *guru* that *kundalini* began to move in a powerful and dramatic manner. The first few weeks after this experience, I felt strong surges up the spine, meditation became easy, and a physical and mental lightness became constant. In the tradition of Yoga, the seeker on the path is advised to prepare himself for *shaktipat* by observing the rules and the regulations as explained by Patanjali in the *Yoga Sutras*. He also practices *asanas, pranayamas* and *mudras* to render the body fit for the impact of strong *shakti* currents. One who is not mentally and emotionally balanced or whose body is not healthy and in tune should not strive for *kundalini* awakening through strenuous methods; he should prepare himself and allow the process to occur when the timing is ideal. There are no mistakes on the *Siddha* Yoga path, for the *guru* is the guide.

We have written of how yogic teachings are imparted according to the need and the aptitude of the seeker. Those who are mild on the path receive general instruction and initiation into simple techniques. Those who are moderate in intent on the path receive advanced instruction. Those who are intense on the path and who are willing to surrender everything that stands in the way of liberation of the Spirit are ideally suited for the *Siddha* Path, the "pure" and direct path.

A *Siddha guru* is one who is a bodily representative of God, as well as a disciple of a *Siddha guru*. Through this line of *gurus*, there flows a current of creative energy or *shakti*, which infiltrates world consciousness and aids in the transformation of material energies. One who is supremely free can function effortlessly on any plane with total realization. Between physical incarnations, such a one either rests in *Siddha-Loka*, the sphere of the masters, or works on some other plane to assist souls seeking liberation from subtle forms of bondage. My great-guru, Sri Yukteswar, after his conscious transition, went to a subtle astral planet to continue his redemptive work, as explained by my *guru* in his book, *Autobiography of a Yogi*. Knowing the universe to be an electrical phenomenon, a perfect master cooperates with the universe and is "in the world but not of it" because of this understanding. The world can be a place of pain and frustration for one who is not awakened, or it can be the stage upon which one can enact the drama of life with understanding. Possessed of inner vision, the *Siddha* master dwells in the consciousness of the highest heaven, regardless of the plane chosen for temporary expression. Mahavatar Babaji once said, "Few people realize that the kingdom of heaven extends fully to this earth plane."

As a result of yogic disciplines and the activity of *shakti*, a master has arrested the decaying process of the body. The descending currents are neutralized by the ascending currents. By neutralizing currents of *prana* in the system, the yogi overcomes death and transcends dualities or opposites. When sun and moon currents are blended, then consciousness takes the route of *sushumna* and flows to the Transcendental Field. The advanced yogi experiences the earth element dissolving into the water element, the water element dissolving into the fire element, the fire element dissolving into the air element, and the air element dissolving into the ether element. With this realization, though he functions within the framework of time, he lives in timelessness. When we understand this state of consciousness, even in part, we can see how certain *Siddha* masters can retain a physical form for centuries of earth time and patiently work with the slowly evolving consciousness of mankind. They can afford to be patient, for they are untouched by time.

Some *Siddha* masters are total renunciates in that they have no family outside of their disciples. Other perfect masters marry and live an outwardly normal life, while maintaining their perfect realization. Whatever role a perfect master plays he plays because it is his cosmic destiny, and he is not in the least influenced by the experience. Whether one's abode is a secluded retreat or a modern house or apartment, what matters is the banishment of ignorance and the inner renunciation of attachments.

It is common for one on the *Siddha* Path eventually to experience, as a result of the upward flow of *kundalini*, the transmutation of sex energy into a more subtle energy, which works to perfect the brain and the nervous system. It is this transmuted energy, along with *shakti*, which imparts radiance and vitality to the body and personality of the accomplished yogi. In the monastic tradition, a seeker on the path is advised to be celibate in order to transmute vital force and to avoid the complications of emotional entanglements. For persons who are married, the advice is to be moderate in sexual relations and to be assured that the mating is ideal and harmonious. In this way, the interchange between male and female energies has a balancing and an elevating influence on the systems of the respective participants.

Throughout the teaching tradition of this path, there is the emphasis that one should always be surrendered to God's will. For one to begin his spiritual quest with the idea of attaining supernatural powers (*siddhis*) is a mistake, for such powers, if expressed through a perfect master, must be spontaneous, with no possibility of egoism involved. Even the desire to emulate the "forever young" or mortal-immortals, while useful as an ideal early on the path, must be renounced if one's destiny is otherwise.

The world of *Siddha* Yoga is far different from any other. It is a reflection of the shining realm beyond *maya*, and one whose intuition is not sufficiently awakened cannot comprehend it. Those who have entered it, however, are assured of conscious immortal life and eventual absorption into the stream of Divine Light.

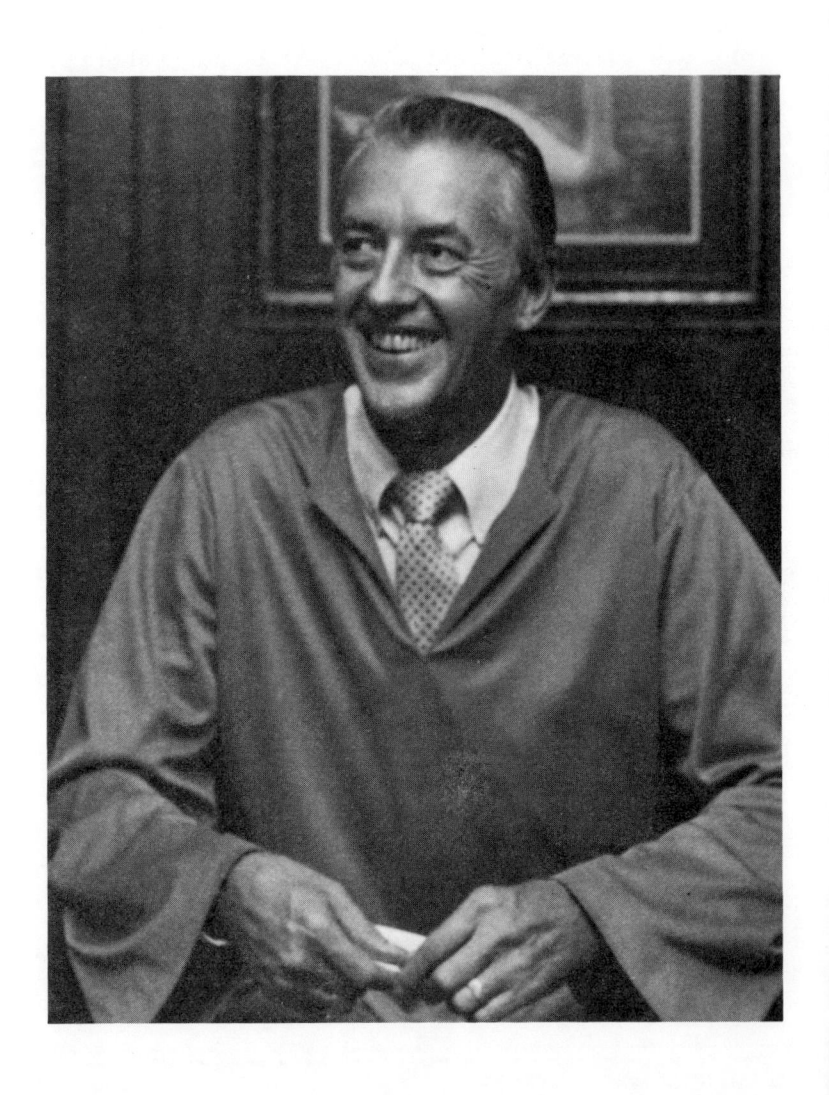

MASTERS OF YOGA

Over the centuries many men and women have awakened to the realization of God and have known the truth about the nature of the world process. Whether all of these persons have practiced specific yogic disciplines or have been impelled from within to yearn for the ultimate experience is beside the point. The fact is that many souls have awakened to the enlightenment experience by one path or another. Most of the examples to follow have been exponents of the practices explained in this book, whether the practices have been intentional or spontaneous. Any approach which leads to Self-Realization can be rightly termed a Yoga path.

Only a few masters of Yoga are here dealt with, some well-known and others not so well-known. The purpose of sharing a little about the experiences and teachings of these persons is to motivate the sincere seeker and give hope to the one who is yet striving on the path that leads from darkness to light. I have made no effort here to determine specific levels of attainment or to assign importance to individual teaching traditions. As all who are in human consciousness share a common awareness, so the enlightened souls share God-Consciousness, regardless of the outer personality characteristics or style of meeting people and the world. It has been my good fortune to know some of the masters of which I write. Others here presented have been an inspiration and a help in many subtle ways during my own *sadhana*.

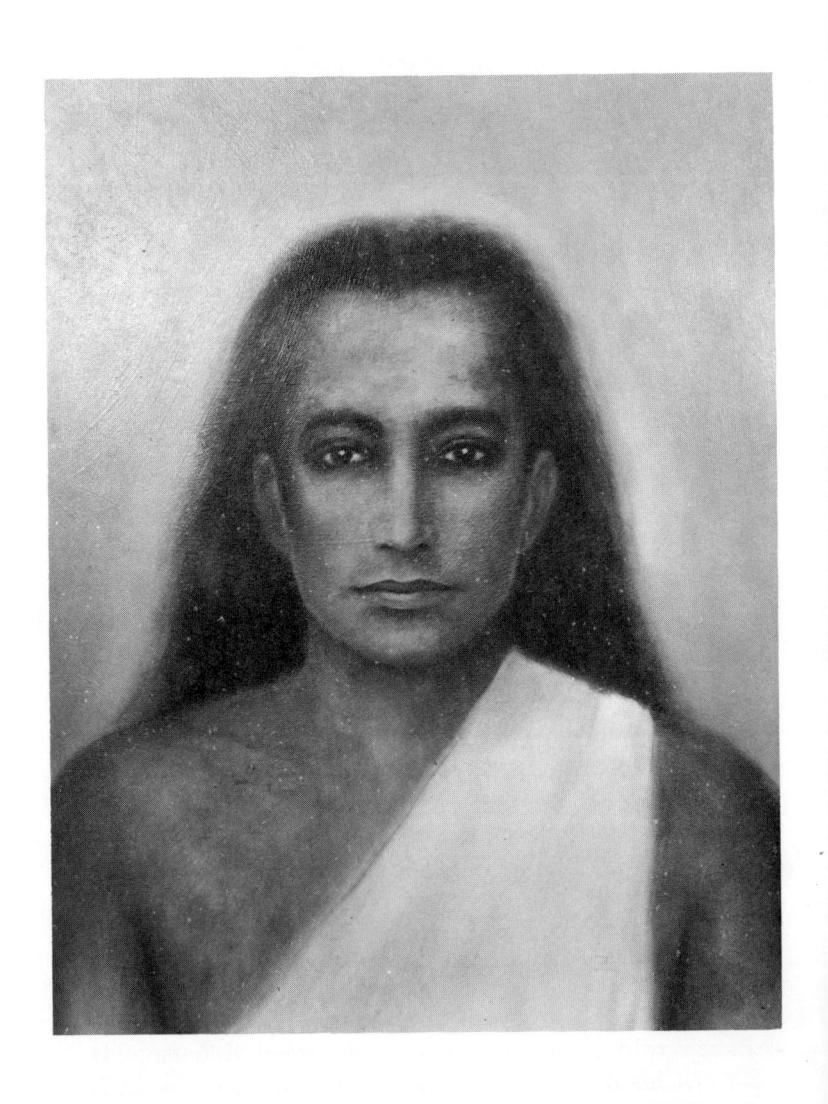

MAHAVATAR BABAJI

For centuries in India, stories have been told of a deathless saint, one of many who are *forever-youthful*, and whose role it is to work with the slow evolutionary trend of planetary consciousness. Very little has been published about this enlightened man known as Babaji, who is considered to be a great *avatar* (*mahavatar*). The reason for our limited public information is that Babaji remains secluded, except for the company of a few advanced disciples whose karmic role it is to be with him in the flesh.

There are now among us several illumined masters who work with the masses. Many of them are spiritually assisted in their mission by Babaji, for it is this master's role to inspire spiritual leaders and to work from the inner planes to uplift human consciousness. While Babaji is best known today as the inspiration behind my line of gurus, he is not limited to this line. Babaji works with any person and any useful spiritual effort to encourage world enlightenment. He is a *Siddha*, a perfected being who has no karmic ties with *maya*, but who is on the earth plane in a physical body to act as a conduit through which the light and power of God can flow into mass consciousness.

Babaji has been embodied for centuries and played the role of Sri Krishna during the time of the great Mahabharata wars in India. The *Bhagavad-Gita* tells of the dialogue between Krishna and his disciple Arjuna and is the text which imparts the profound philosophical treatise upon which the science of Yoga is based. Babaji told Lahiri Mahasaya and Swami Kebalananda, two of his disciples, of how he initiated Shankara (A.D. 788-820) into the science of *Kriya Yoga* in Benaras (now Varnarasi). Shankara's historically known guru was Govinda Jati. Other Yoga masters initiated by Babaji in time past are known to be Kabir and some of the masters who wrote the basic texts detailing the practices as explained in the first part of this book. It can be said that wherever there is a yogic tradition which stresses *kriyas*, practiced intentionally or experienced spontaneously, Babaji's influence is pronounced.

Babaji himself has used *kriya pranayama* to maintain his body through dynamic *kundalini* activity and an infusion of cosmic energy. Though using a body, he is cosmic conscious, and his physical form merely serves as a focus for his work on this plane. In the tradition of all enlightened masters, Babaji teaches according to temperament and the capacity of the seeker, giving useful guidelines for responsible living to the average seeker and initiating into advanced *kriyas* those who are ready for more dramatic change in consciousness. Because he has no subtle mental impression (*vasanas*) to restrict his consciousness, this great master is on earth only because of Divine will, that mankind might be beneficially influenced.

Avatars play their roles according to the need in the cosmic drama, and Babaji's role is that of an *avatar* of *Shiva*. His mission is to work with planetary consciousness during this transition from the Dark Age to the Age of Enlightenment, to aid in the acceleration of mankind's awakening to spiritual values and to neutralize somewhat the stress and strain of misguided human activities. There are also certain celestial and planetary influences which must be worked with in this current cycle. These influences require the presence on earth of illumined masters who serve to direct some of the energies in harmony with the evolutionary trend. The work of enlightened masters on earth, as well as on subtle planes, is our assurance that the Divine pattern will unfold in line with the inherent intention.

Babaji resided in Northern India during the last century, in the mountain area near Badrinarayan, not far from the border of Nepal. It was in this area, on Drongiri Mountain near Ranikhet, that Babaji initiated Lahiri Mahasaya into *Kriya Yoga* and asked his disciple to return to his community to teach others the sacred science. This took place in the autumn of 1861. At the *Kumbha Mela* (major religious gathering of laymen and saints) held at Allahabad, where the Ganges, Jamuna and Saraswati rivers come together, Swami Sri Yukteswar met Babaji (1894) and was instructed by him to write his masterly treatise, *The Holy Science*. Several close disciples of Lahiri Mahasaya had personal contact with Babaji over the years, either by association with him in the Himalayas or due to Babaji's appearance to them in a vision or in his light body.

Because he has been known by so many people for many centuries, Babaji's personal history is unknown. We have said that he played the role of Sri Krishna, and it is certain that he was known by other names in different centuries. Some of the titles of respect given him by Lahiri Mahasaya's disciples are Mahamuni Babaji Maharaj (Supreme Ecstatic Master), Maha Yogi (the Great Yogi), and Trambak Baba or Shiva Baba (titles denoting *avatars* of *Shiva*). There is some evidence to connect him with a more recent appearance of a great saint known as Sri Hairakhan Baba, of which more will be told in a later segment of this text.

My guru has written an extensive account of Babaji, which appears in his *Autobiography of a Yogi,* and has told personal disciples that Babaji renews his body every several decades through a unique yogic process. The master sometimes appears youthful and sometimes more mature, sometimes clean shaven and sometimes with mustache or beard. No matter what the outer appearance, Babaji is ever the same as a conscious free spirit.

As the initiator of several masters of Yoga, Babaji has infused his realization and cosmic knowledge into many of the great spiritual traditions. He is also known to conduct personally special ceremonies involving *mantras* and other practices, designed to invite intelligent energies into the earth sphere for the purpose of quickening planetary evolution.

When Paramahansa Yogananda prepared to leave India to come to America in 1920, he prayed for Babaji's blessing. After a time spent in prayer and meditation, Babaji came to Yoganandaji's home in Calcutta and talked with him. He said: "You are the one I have chosen to spread the message of *Kriya Yoga* in the West. Long ago I met your guru Yukteswar at a *Kumbha Mela;* I told him then I would send you to him for training. *Kriya Yoga* will ultimately spread to all lands and aid in harmonizing the nations through man's personal, transcendental perception of the Infinite God."

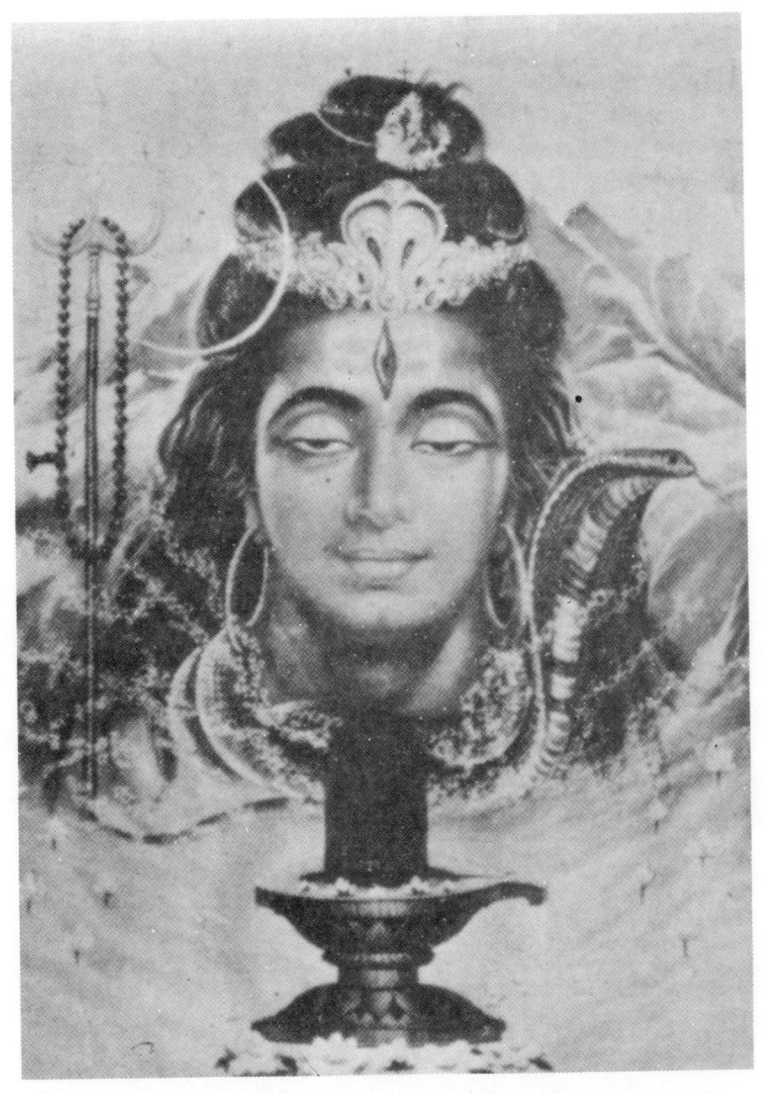

God is the aspect of Lord Shiva; the aspect which forms the worlds and then dissolves them. Shiva's third eye is open, the serpent represents wisdom, a *shivalinga* (Symbol of Shiva's cosmic activity) is in the front. *From a painting.*

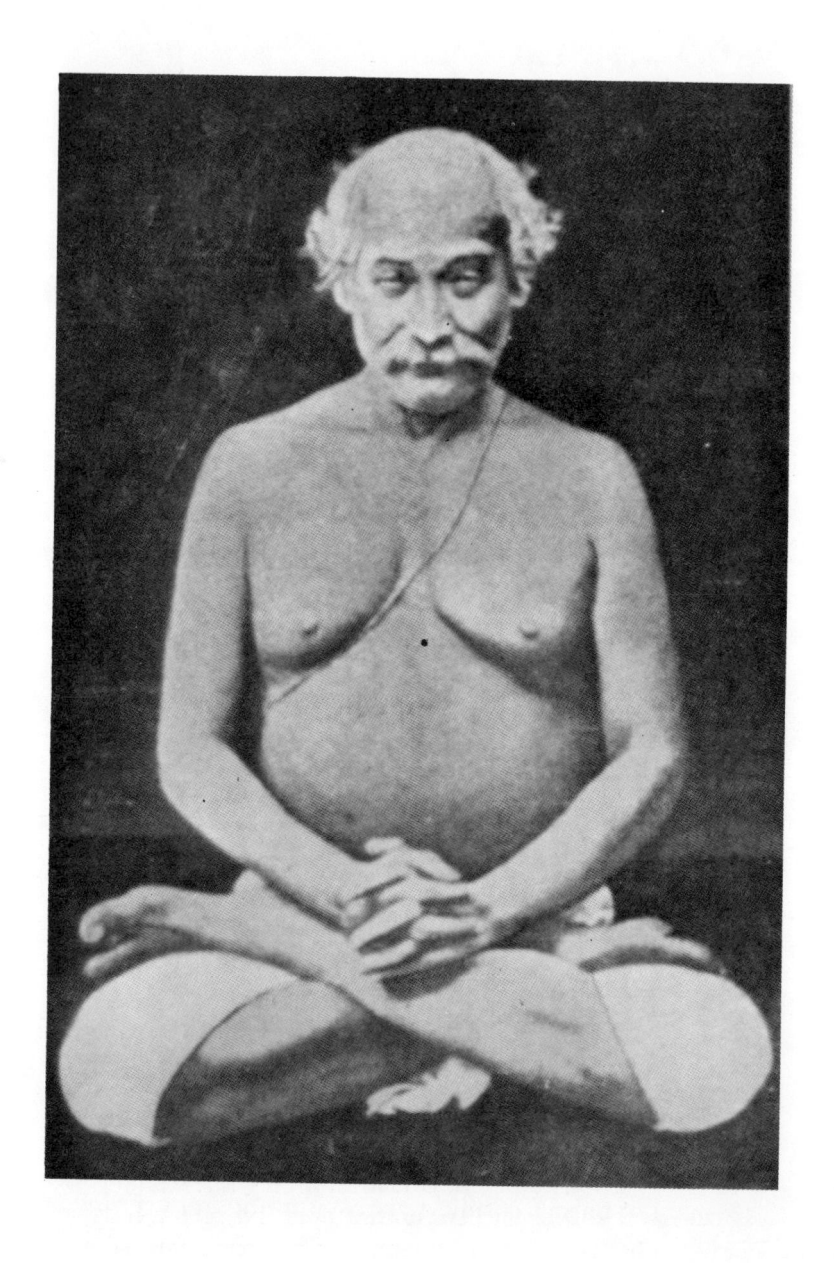

YOGAVATAR LAHIRI MAHASAYA

In accord with the trend of the new era, there was born in India, in 1828, a man who was to play a decided role in introducing the science of *Kriya Yoga* to the world. In the village of Ghurni, in the district of Nadia in Bengal, Shyamacharan Lahiri, as a young boy, would often meditate and seek out quiet places for contemplation. His family was devoted to God in the aspect of *Shiva* and built several temples for the purpose of private and public worship of this manifestation.

At school in Vanarasi, Lahiri was exposed to various languages including English, Sanskrit, Urdu, Hindi, Bengali and some Persian. Possessed of great vitality, he was active in sports and would often swim in the Ganges River. At eighteen he was married to Kashimoni Devi, who later became his disciple and was intitiated into yogic practices. Two sons were born of this union. Both Tinkari and Dukari Lahiri followed in their father's tradition of *Kriya Yoga* meditation.

Lahiri Mahasaya, as he became known to disciples, accepted a job as a clerk for the Military Works Branch. This department had the duty of supplying materials for the army's road building projects. He also taught Hindi, Urdu and Bengali to various engineers and officers of his department. While practicing yogic methods in the privacy of his home, Lahiri attended to his family duties and social obligations. In this manner, he became an example to others that it is possible to live a normal life and still attain the highest goal of Self-Realization.

In 1861 (a close relative of Lahiri's states 1868), Lahiri was transferred to Ranikhet, a forest region near Nainital in the Himalayas. One afternoon while wandering about the Dronigiri mountain area, he met a holy man who addressed him by name: "Shyamacharan, you have come!" The holy man was Babaji, who had chosen the occasion to renew the guru-disciple relationship which had been theirs for several incarnations. Lahiri was taken to a cave and shown the simple belongings of a recluse: a water pot, meditation staff and other items, which he recalled as being his after Babaji awakened his inner vision with a simple blessing. With a single touch, an electric current passed through Lahiri's brain, enabling him to know of his true relationship with Babaji and of his previous experiences as a mountain yogi. Babaji informed his disciple that the *Kriya Yoga* path was really his own, because one of Lahiri's ancestors was the great sage Shandilya. The *Shandilya Upanishad* predates Patanjali's *Yoga-Sutras*.

In seven days Lahiri was instructed in the complete process of *Kriya Yoga* and various procedures. After this preliminary instruction, Babaji gave him some oil to drink, which further purified his body. Then initiation into *Kriya Yoga* was given, after which Lahiri spent seven days in unbroken *samadhi*. The momentum of previous spiritual disciplines and the grace of his guru enabled Lahiri to master in a short time that which takes several lifetimes for the average seeker on the path. In fact, Lahiri was liberated in his previous incarnation and came when he did in a new body to set an example for a seeking world—to show the possibilities available to all who would live an orderly life and meditate on God.

While with Babaji, the newly awakened Lahiri had occasion to observe several interesting incidents. One of them occurred when he visited a temple a few miles away and observed at night a holy man coming to worship there. A bright halo surrounded this holy man, whom Babaji said was the son of Dronacharya. The preceptor Dronacharya, of *Mahabharata* times, once lived at this place with the *Pandavas*, who were part of the epic struggle going on at the time. His son, like Babaji, is considered to be a *mortal-immortal*.

Before leaving Ranikhet, Lahiri initiated a few disciples into *Kriya Yoga* practice. It was characteristic of him to share the techique with almost all who came to him with a sincere desire for spiritual unfoldment. People of all religious faiths were initiated over the years. With Lahiri, the age-old restrictions concerning yogic initiation were relaxed somewhat, as Babaji agreed that, in the current era, Yoga should be taught to a wider number of persons and not just to the few who could live in a retreat environment.

The master taught his disciples to live in the world with understanding and to continue their spiritual practices faithfully. Highly advanced yogis were also initiated by Lahiri Mahasaya, including Swami Sri Yukteswar, Swami Pranavananda, Keshavananda Avadhut, Sri Shastri Mahasaya, Srimat Bhupendranath, Dayal Maharaj and Ram Gopal. So highly respected was he that Lahiri was once mentioned by the great renunciate **Swami Trailanga**, who said of him: "I have renounced all for that which Lahiri has been given by God."

Twenty-two publications, commentaries on various scriptures were the result of Lahiri Mahasaya's efforts to bring the message of God-Realization to the average person. A disciple, Panchanan Bhattacharya, assisted greatly in the recording and publishing of these works.

Kriya Yoga methods as taught by Lahiri were streamlined and simplified for use by ordinary seekers. The essential techniques he taught form the basis for a regular practice, which can awaken latent forces in a true seeker and be the means of liberation of consciousness. While he made no effort to form an organization during his lifetime, he knew one would come into being. (In fact, several different groups represent his teaching emphasis, as a result of his various disciples becoming gurus in their own right.) The major public outreach was to find expression through Swami Sri Yukteswar, who founded two Yoga training ashrams and prepared Paramahansa Yogananda for his mission in the West. When Yoganandaji was a year old, his father, who was a disciple of Lahiri, took him to the great guru. Lahiri held

Yoganandaji on his lap and said: "He will be a great engine and bring many souls to God."

A true incarnation of Yoga (*yogavatar*) comes for a specific purpose into this world and leaves when his mission is fulfilled. Thus it was that Babaji told Sri Yukteswar, at their 1894 meeting at the *Kumbha Mela,* to pass Lahiri a message to the effect that the *Yogavatar's* time to experience *mahasamadhi* was not far off. Six months before his transition, Lahiri told his wife of his plans to depart during the month of September 1895. On the 26th of that month, which was *Mahastami,* the second day of worship for the divine Mother as *Durga,* a ritual ceremony was being conducted in the home of a neighbor of the Lahiri's. In this ritual, the most significant moment is at the transition of the phase of the moon, as it gets brighter from the eighth to ninth day. At this moment Lahiri Mahasaya opened his eyes for a moment, then closed them to retire into deeper meditation and made his conscious exist from the body. Three close disciples, who were not present, had a vision of Lahiri at the time he was making his conscious *samadhi.* The following day, after the body had been cremated at the Manikarnika Ghat by the Ganges, another disciple, Swami Keshabananda, was in his room when a great light filled the space. Lahiri Mahasaya appeared as flesh and blood, younger and more radiant in appearance. He said to his disciple: "My householder work in the world is done; but I do not leave the earth entirely. Henceforth I shall spend some time with Babaji in the Himalayas, and with Babaji in the cosmos."

Some illumined beings continue their redemptive work for the world after leaving their physical form by working through a body of light. In this way they infuse the consciousness of the planet with useful energy, as well as work on the inner planes with receptive disciples. Those close to Lahiri's wife have said that in later years, after he had left his body, he would enter her private room while she meditated and would converse with her.

JNANAVATAR SRI YUKTESWAR

It is interesting to note how different masters express various facets of *yogic* attainment. Because he is best known for his characteristic insight into the nature of Consciousness, Sri Yukteswar (the monastic name means union with *Isvara*) can be referred to as an Incarnation of Knowledge, a *Jnanavatar*. He entered the monastic order of Swamis, after the death of his wife, and devoted the rest of his life to training disciples at his two ashrams, one at Puri and the other at Serampore, near Calcutta.

Born Priya Nath Karar in 1855 of wealthy parents, this master of Yoga spent his adult years managing family properties and undertaking the responsibilities of husband and father. In his middle years, he met his *guru*, Lahiri Mahasaya, and devoted himself to the practice of *Kriya Yoga*. His formal initiation into the Swami Order took place at Buddh Gaya in Bengal.

Sri Yukteswar was also an astrologer of repute and a master of Ayurvedic knowledge, concerning the uses of gems and metals worn on the body for therapeutic purposes. He also researched the Cosmic Cycles *(yugas)* and found an error in the Hindu almanac and thereby proved his theory of the 24,000 year equinoctial major cycle (during which sub-cycles of 4800 years, 3600 years, 2400 years and 1200 years were manifest). These years are the: Golden Age, Mental Age, Electrical Age and Dark Age, respectively, with 12,000 being the number of descending years and 12,000 being the number of ascending years. This explanation is set forth in his slim book, *The Holy Science* (*Kaivalya Darsanam*), which he wrote at the request of Babaji after their initial meeting at Allahabad in 1894. I have also discussed Sri Yukteswar's conclusions regarding the Cosmic Cycles in my book, *The Way of the Initiate*.

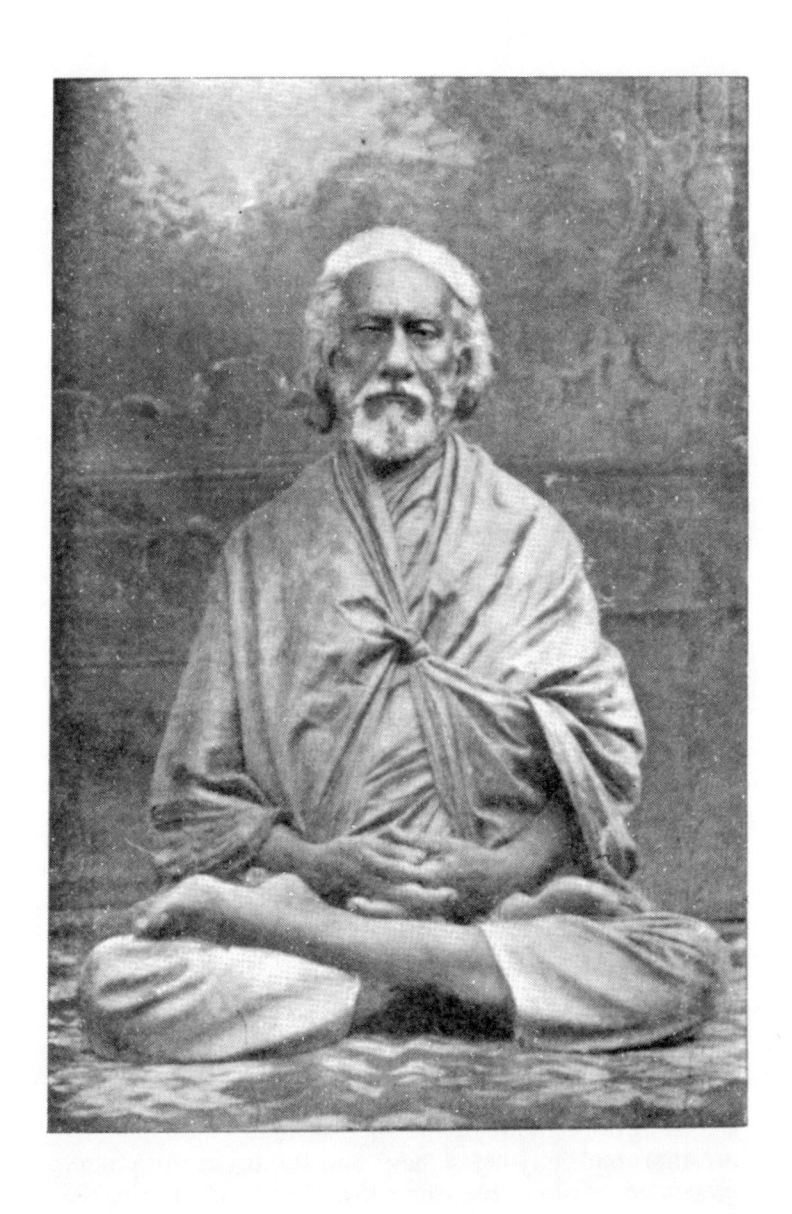

Known to disciples as an adept in the spiritual healing arts, Sri Yukteswar never openly displayed his *siddhis* but preferred to work quietly and without public notice. He was extremely practical, and, when Yoganandaji, as a young man, thought of forsaking his family relationships, Sri Yukteswar counseled: "Why exclude relatives from your love of humanity?" He also exhibited the ability to visit disciples in a subtle body and to appear to them in visions in time of need. He had only a few disciples. Yoganandaji once said, "My *guru* could have been the most sought after *guru* in India if it were not for his strict training of disciples." Another time, when a visitor looked at a portrait of Sri Yukteswar and mentioned that he appeared to be a fine man, Yoganandaji exclaimed with awe in his voice: "He was no man, he was a god!"

Paramahansa Yogananda was trained for ten years in his *guru's* ashram before being sent to the West in 1920. At that time Yukteswar said: "Go now and all doors will open to you." He showed a keen interest in the work of his major disciple, and they carried on correspondence over the years. In 1935, in Los Angeles, California, Yoganandaji had a vision of his *guru,* in which Sri Yukteswar bade him to return to India, because he planned to enter *mahasamadhi* before long.

On March 9, 1936, the great master made his conscious departure from the body and was buried in the garden of his Puri ashram, where a memorial temple now stands. Three months later, in his room in a Bombay hotel, Yoganandaji saw and conversed with Sri Yukteswar in his resurrected form. He gave personal information about world trends, explained in detail about life in the subtle realms and informed his disciple that he was presently active as a savior to advanced souls on an astral planet, Hiranyaloka. There most inhabitants are withdrawing from astral attachments in preparation for more subtle realms. The Amrita Bazar Patrika, a newspaper of Calcutta, carried the following story after the burial of Sri Yuketswar's physical form:

"One of the great expounders of the *Bhagavad-Gita*, Swami Maharaj was a great disciple of Yogiraj Sri Shyama Charan Lahiri Mahasaya of Benaras. Swami Maharaj was the founder of several Yogoda Satsanga centers in India, and was the great inspiration behind the yoga movement which was carried to the West by Swami Yogananda, his principle disciple. It was Sri Yukteswarji's prophetic powers and deep realization that inspired Swami Yogananda to cross the oceans and spread in America the message of the masters of India. His interpretations of the *Bhagavad-Gita* and other scriptures testify to the depth of Sri Yukteswarji's command of the philosophy, both Eastern and Western, and remain as an eye-opener for the unity between Orient and Occident. As he believed in the unity of all religious faiths, Sri Yukteswar Maharaj established the Sadhu Sabba (Society of Saints) with the cooperation of leaders of various sects and faiths, for the inculcation of a scientific spirit in religion. At the time of his demise he nominated Swami Yogananda his successor as the president of Sadhu Sabha. India is really poorer today by the passing of such a great man. May all fortunate enough to have come near him inculcate in themselves the true spirit of India's culture and *sadhana* which was personified in him."

Many of the centers established by Sri Yukteswar have been incorporated into the Self-Realization Fellowship movement and continue to spread *Kriya Yoga* to thousands in India, as well as now to provide schools and clinics. Other disciples of his have established ashrams, through which the teaching tradition has flowed for decades, without association with any major organized effort. The writings of Sri Yukteswar were influential in making clear many points which are to be found in chapter two of this book. He is not only presently active in subtle realms but is also influential through his inspired life in making possible a more comprehensive understanding for those who seek in this tradition.

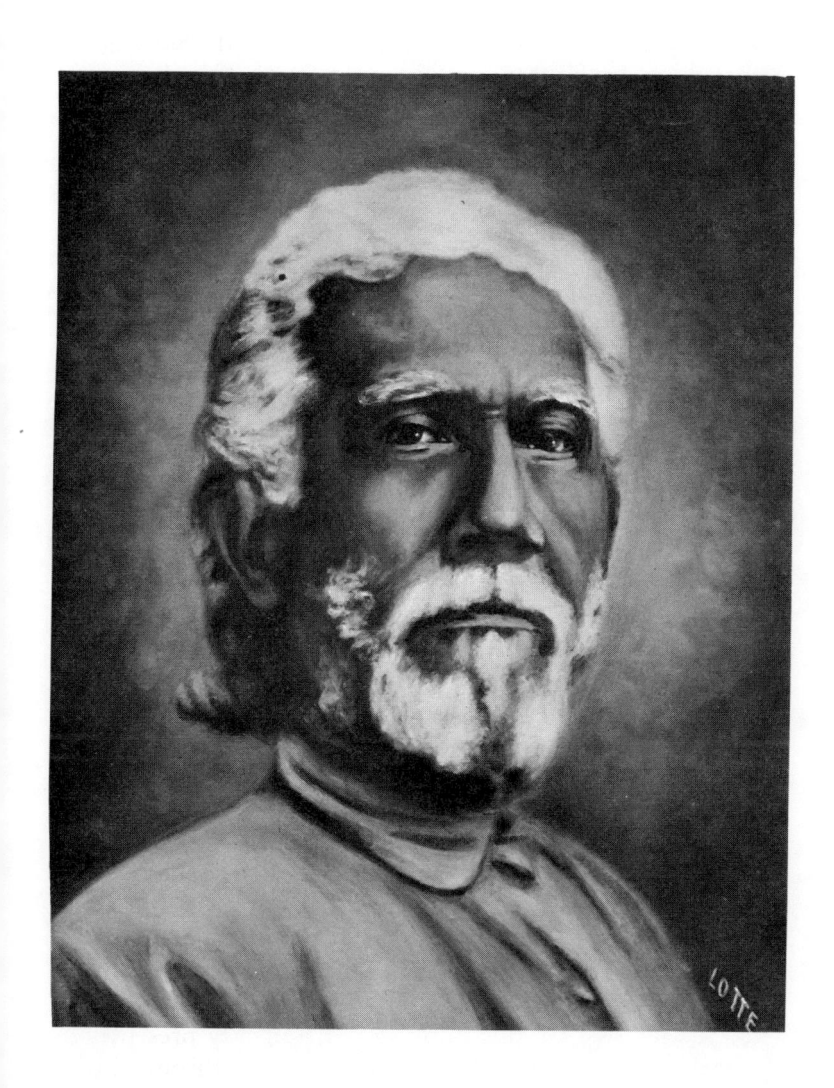

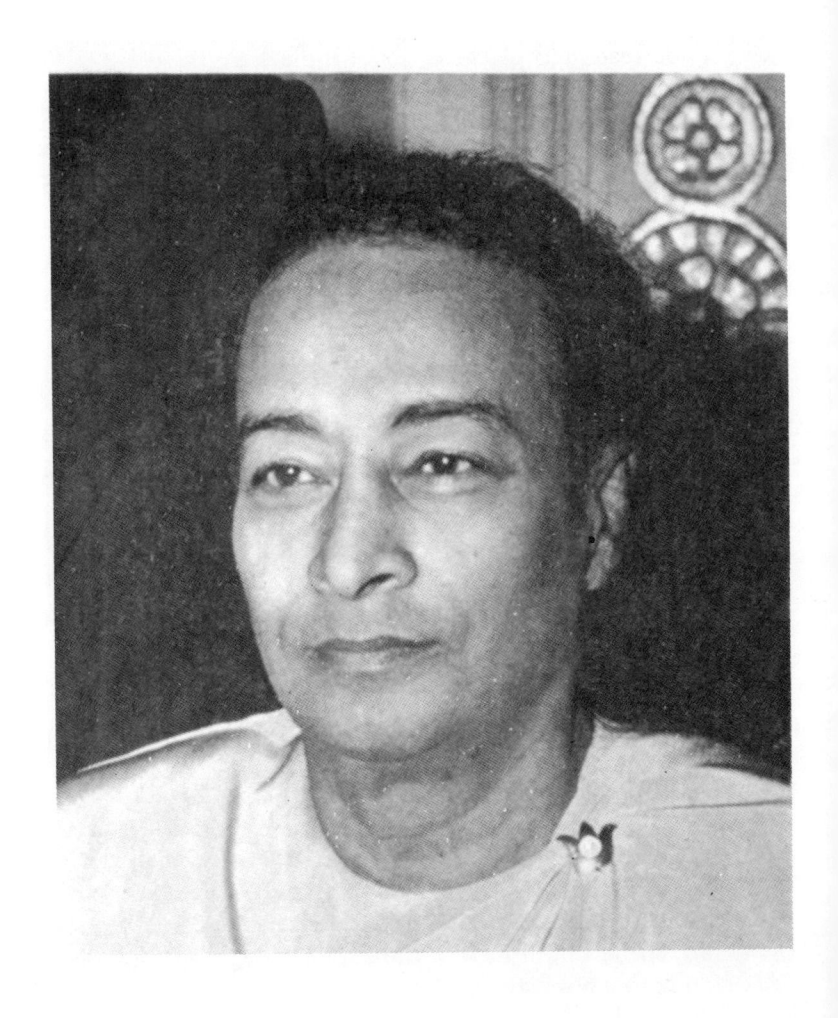

PREMAVATAR PARAMAHANSA YOGANANDA

The teachings of the yogis of India were known to a few in America in the early part of this century, but it was Paramahansa Yogananda who brought Yoga to the West in dramatic and practical fashion.

Born Mukunda Lal Ghose on January 5, 1893, in Gorakhpur in northeastern India near the Himalaya Mountains, he was one of eight children born to his parents, both of whom were disciples of Lahiri Mahasaya. As a boy, he grew up in relative comfort, since his father was an executive of one of the railroad companies and commanded a substantial salary. Baptized by Lahiri Mahasaya at the age of one year, the young Mukunda often visited saints and masters as he grew up, learning from them the secret science behind Yoga and being impelled on the path of awakening. He told us that he was conscious while in his mother's womb and recalled many of his previous incarnations as a yogi in the Himalayan mountains.

At the age of twelve, he once entered his attic meditation room in the family home at Calcutta and was absorbed in *samadhi* for forty-eight hours, during which time he experienced the manifestation and the dissolution of the universe and roamed in the higher heavens *(lokas)*. Yoganandaji told us that he came for the express purpose of teaching Yoga in the West and that it was Babaji's intention that he do so. Even as Babaji had summoned Lahiri Mahasaya back to the earth plane for the purpose of setting an example to people of the world, so he summoned Yoganandaji to be a missionary of Yoga to a waiting world.

As a college student, Yogananda met his *guru* Swami Sri Yukteswar, and spent ten years in the most exacting training under him. Few could have withstood the strict discipline but, then, Yoganandaji was not an ordinary seeker on the path. He had come on a mission, and his training under Sri Yukteswar, who had a keen interest in world enlightenment, provided the needed emphasis and direction for his work. After receiving his college education, Mukunda Lal Ghose became Swami Yogananda (July 1914) by virtue of being initiated into that venerable monastic order. Like Sri Yukteswar, he became a member of the mountain *(giri)* branch of the Order. *Ananda* means "bliss", and Yogananda means "the bliss of Yoga" or "bliss through Yoga." Yogananda is a fairly common monastic name among swamis.

Before coming to America, Yoganandaji took part in the organizational work instituted by his *guru* and founded a school at Ranchi for the education of children. A feature at this school was and is the practice of *Yogasanas* and meditation. While meditating one day, Yoganandaji had a vision in which he saw a vast number of people and knew they were disciples yet to be met in America. He was invited to Boston to speak at a religious conference and, through the generous financial assistance of his father, was able to remain in modest circumstances after the conference was over.

In Boston he accepted his first American disciples and began to teach classes. Before long he was to tour the major cities speaking to audiences who packed the auditoriums. Wherever he went, he was hosted by leading citizens, including business leaders, mayors, governors and even the President of the United States (Calvin Coolidge, 1927). After laying the foundation by much traveling, Yoganandaji settled in Southern California and purchased, with the aid of disciples, a large estate in the suburbs of Los Angeles. This location, Mount Washington Estates, still serves as the international headquarters for Self-Realization Fellowship, which he founded.

Yoganandaji's ideal was to present a practical message and to teach with the aim of both quantity and quality in mind: quantity to reach the masses with a helpful philosophy and quality in personal work with receptive disciples. He often said that many of his disciples had been with him before, when he lived in India in his previous incarnation, and had come back to work out their liberation and to assist him in spreading the work.

His only return visit to India was in 1935-36, and it was then that Sri Yukteswar gave him the further title *Paramahansa,* which is the highest title to be given to a yogi. *Hansa* means "swan," and popular belief is that a swan can drink a mixture of milk and water, taking only the milk from the mixture. Thus, a *paramahansa* is a "high swan" among yogis, who can live in the world and extract only the Divine essence.

Upon his return to America, Yoganandji was presented with a hermitage retreat at Encinitas, California, a gift of his chief disciple James J. Lynn (Rajarsi Janakananda), who was a millionaire businessman as well as an advanced yogi. In the early part of the fourth decade, Yoganandaji founded two churches, one in Hollywood and another in San Diego. He named each a "Church of All Religions" and alternated Sunday services between them for several years. Ten years later, an addition was built on the Hollywood Church site, and a new shrine was dedicated at Pacific Palisades, California.

While his California work was progressing over the years, his organization sent Yoga lessons to thousands of seekers through the mail. His *Autobiography of a Yogi,* published in 1946, took the word to additional thousands and is now published in fourteen major world languages. It is estimated that over 100,000 persons received *Kriya Yoga* initiation from him during his ministry in the West, which spanned thirty-two years.

In 1950, Yoganandaji retired from public work and secluded himself at his desert retreat near Twenty-Nine Palms, California, to write an extensive commentary on the *Bhagavad-Gita* and other scriptures. It was at this time that I met him, and I have told of this experience in my book, *Darshan: The Vision of Light.*

In the months preceding his *mahasamadhi,* he informed us that his work was finished and that he was planning to leave us. He had established the organization on a sound financial basis and had trained key disciples to carry on in his spirit, thus proving to be a master of organizational detail as well as a master of Yoga. He told us he would rest for a while in subtle realms, then return to the earth plane to be with Babaji in the Himalayas.

On March 7, 1952, after delivering a short talk to a special gathering of devotees and representatives of India (including India's Ambassador), he lifted his eyes and passed into *mahasamadhi*. Years before he had said to disciples: "When I go, I want to go with my boots on, speaking of God and the great Masters." His wish was fulfilled. A few weeks later, Forest Lawn Mortuary officials sent a notarized letter to the Self-Realization Fellowship officers stating that Yoganandaji's physical body had not shown any evidence of decay, even though several weeks had passed before it was placed in a crypt there. Yogis have long taught that the correct practice of *Kriya Yoga* actually purifies and transforms even the physical body.

Through the continued ministry of the Self-Realization Fellowship and the independent works of other direct disciples, Paramahansa Yogananda's energy and teaching tradition persists. He prophesied that the work would grow after his passing and be a major influence for good in the world. To disciples who asked him about the *guru-disciple* attunement after his passing, he said: "If you think me near, I will be near."

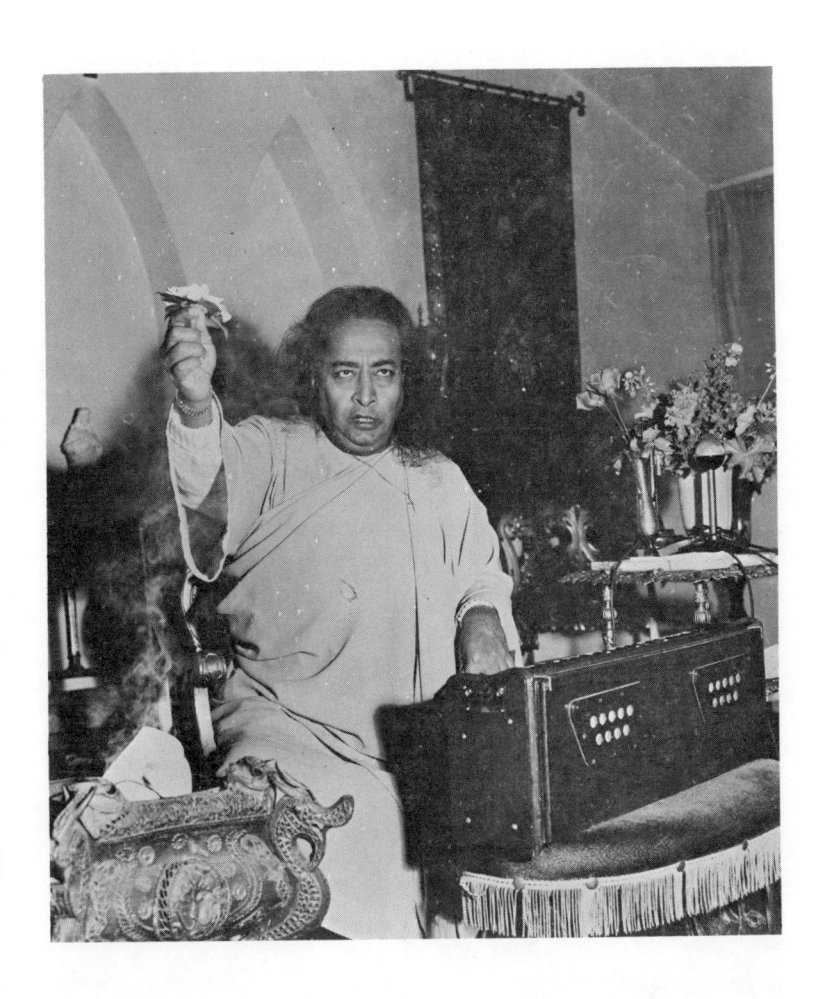

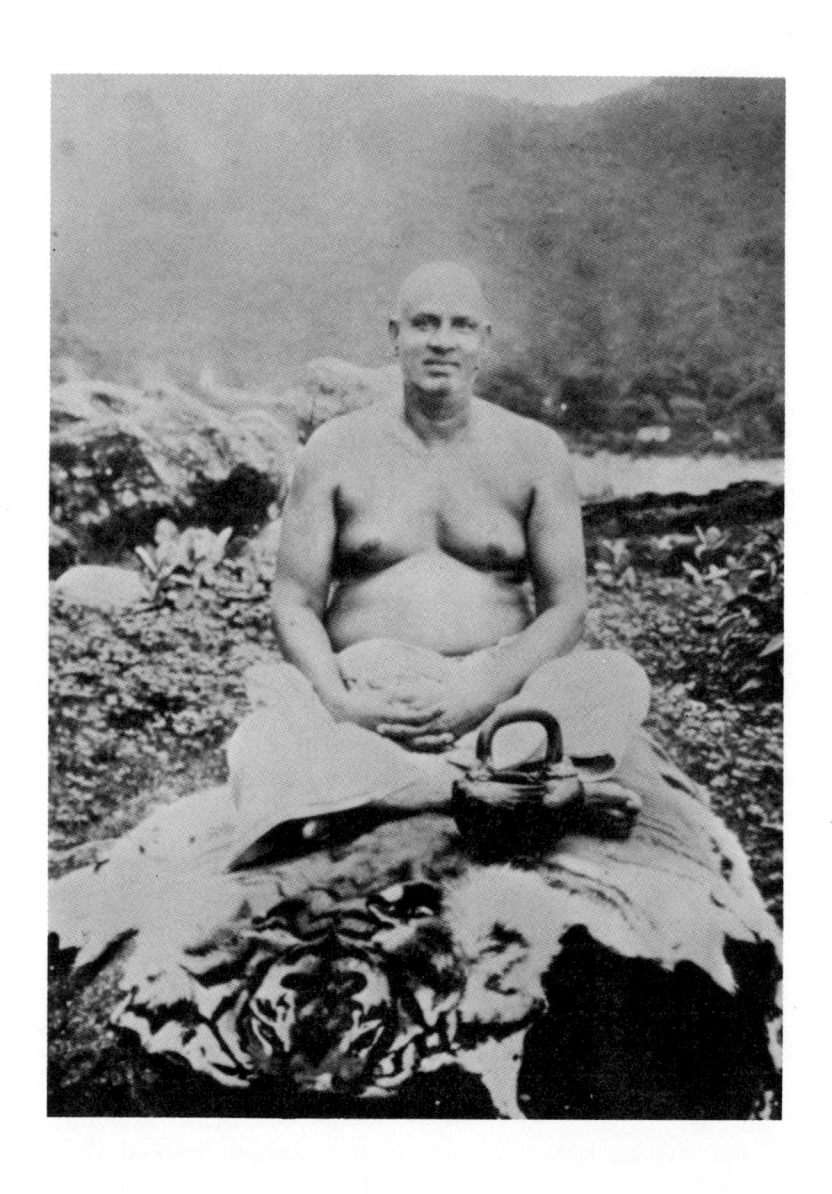

SWAMI SIVANANDA SARASWATI

Swami Sivananda is known the world over as one of the leaders in the tradition of Yoga. He was born in Pattamadia, near Tirunelveli, in Tamil Nadu, on September 8, 1887, and was named Kuppuswami. As a boy, he would gather flowers for his father's daily ceremonial worship of *Shiva* and then listen to the *Vedic* recitations and the scriptural readings. He joined in family prayers and sang devotional songs.

After High School, he enrolled in the Tanjore Medical Institute and, before long, began to publish a monthly magazine devoted to advising readers on Ayurvedic medicine. As a doctor, Kuppuswami went to Singapore and there practiced the healing arts. He was loved by almost all with whom he came into contact and moved freely in society. He was known to be a student of philosophy and encouraged his peers and patients to sing devotional songs.

Returning to India, he went to Rishikesh, the holy city where a great many monks make their abode. There, in 1924, he became Swami Sivananda Saraswati, as a result of receiving initiation from his guru, Swami Viswananda. The next several years were spent in severe discipline and inner research through yogic practices. Sivanandaji also ministered to the health needs of the other renunciates and began to collect money for the purpose of printing and free distribution of tracts and booklets dealing with the higher life. In the early 1930's, an ashram, which became known as the Divine Life Society, began to grow up around this dynamic monk. As years went on, it became one of the largest and the farthest reaching of any ashram devoted to yogic practices. Magazines and books began to pour from the ashram presses, and at least as many copies were given away free as were sold through dealers. The Swami himself authored over two hundred books in his lifetime.

In the tradition of world teachers, Sivanandaji welcomed all to his fold and taught the message of universal brotherhood and the love of God. He taught that service to humanity was as important to one on the path as meditation and inner exploration. Many Americans and Europeans, who heard of Sivanandaji's work and wrote him a letter, were often surprised to receive, by airmail, a personal letter and a parcel of books free of any charge.

In the tradition of great Yoga masters, this exalted soul passed from his body consciously on July 14, 1963, at 11:15 P.M., in harmony with favorable planetary influences, during the final phase of the northern solstice.

The Divine Life Ashram at Rishikesh remains a center of light and learning under the inspired influence of Sivanandaji's chosen disciple, Swami Chidananda. Many other disciples have been trained by Sivanandaji and sent to various places in the world to teach. Swami Satchidananda, who founded the Integral Yoga Institute, is well-known, as is Swami Vishnudevananda of Canada and the Bahamas. Divine Life Centers and branches are in many parts of India, as well as South America, Switzerland, Canada, the United States, South America, Australia, Malaysia, Mauritius, Ceylon and Trinidad.

How does the light from one man shine so bright and inspire so many millions on the path? Swami Sivananda would say it is due to God's grace and the creative impulse of the Divine Energy, which flows forth to meet the deepest yearnings of seeking souls. Swamiji was a perfect blend of yogic science and practical application of creative principles. In every project his motto was, "Do it now!"

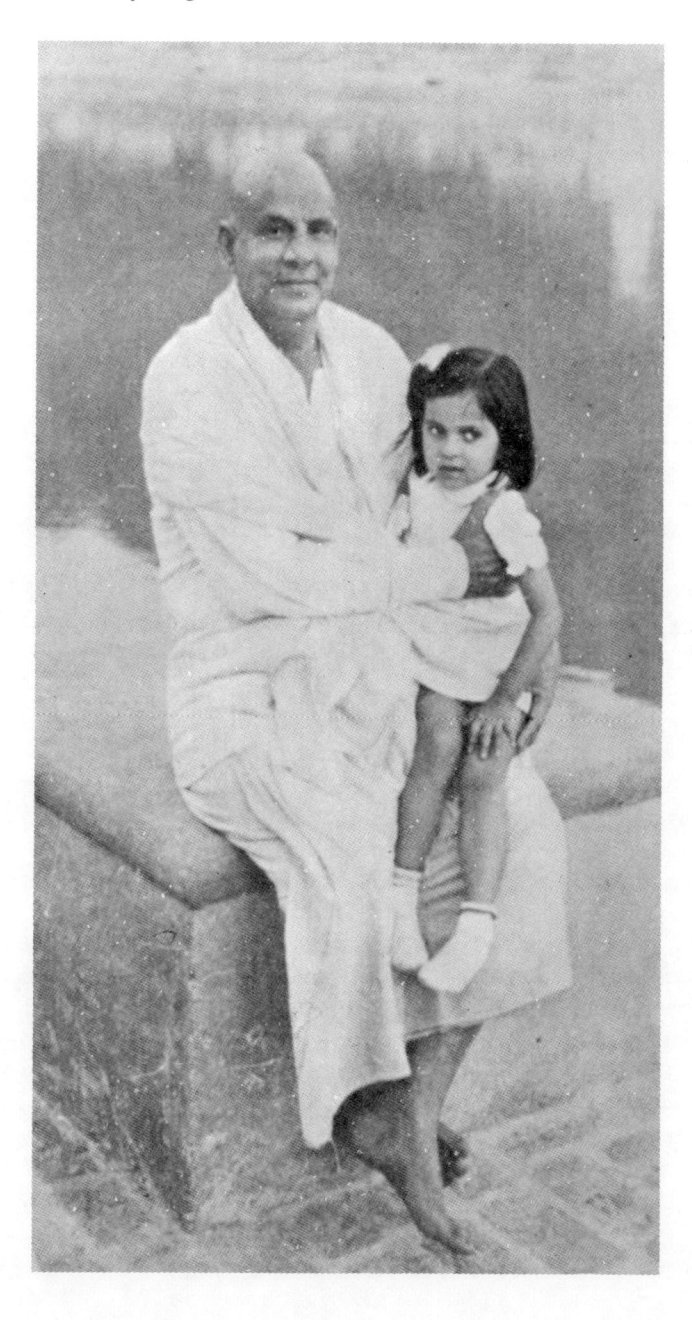

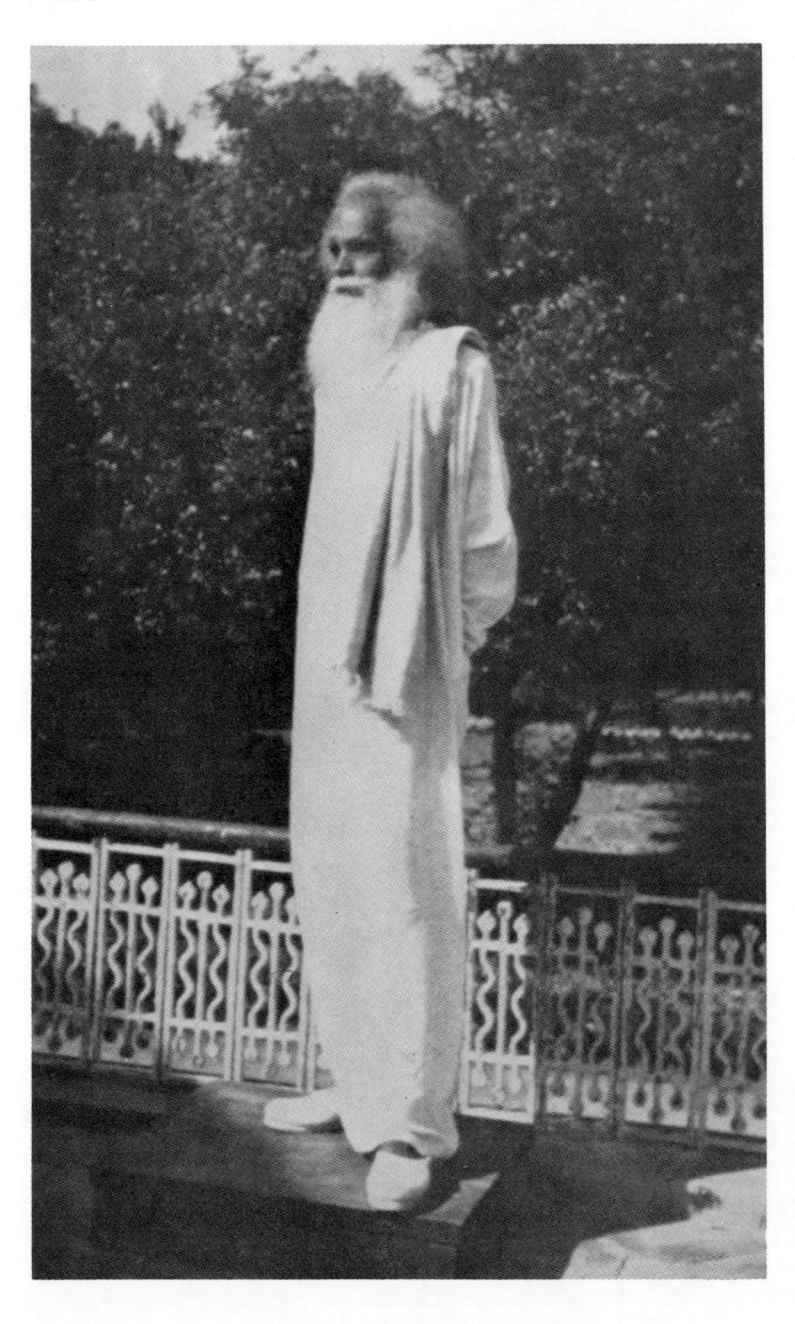

SHIVAPURI BABA

One of the more inspiring stories is that of a modern saint who lived his life almost unknown to the outside world, until John G. Bennett presented the drama through his masterly book, *Long Pilgrimage*. In this book is told the amazing experiences and practical teachings of Govinda Bharati, later known as Shivapuri Baba, so named because he chose as his residence the Shivapuri Forest in Nepal during the final years of his earth incarnation. When he passed consciously in 1963, he was 137 years of age.

Born in 1826 of a Brahmin family in the State of Kerala, as one of a set of twins (the other child was a girl), Govinda was believed by his grandfather, who was an astrologer, to be a great *sannyasin* whose life would fulfill the purpose of the family line. At the age of eighteen, the young Govinda renounced the world and followed his grandfather into the forest, there to be trained in the scriptures and to learn the secret sciences of the Vedic seers.

Before his own death, the grandfather told his charge that he had left a fortune in diamonds and other precious stones for Govinda's use in the world after he had attained God-Realization. The young man was told that it would be his duty to make a pilgrimage around the world, and it was for this reason that financial plans were laid for the future.

At Shankaramutt in southern India, the young renunciate was initiated and took the name of Govindananda Bharati. He later was to say that initiation was not really necessary for him, but he did it as an act of religious devotion to traditional ideals. He next moved into the Narbada Forest, protected from chance visitors by an impenetrable jungle. There, living on natural foods, he remained, with the intention of following the path of *Itambhara Prajna* or Absolute Realization of God beyond all forms and images. This is attained as one leaves behind every support and comfort of the mind. We are told the sage lost track of relative time as years passed, and over thirty years was spent on the inner quest before Govinda came back to social contacts.

True to his renunciate ideals, he would never discuss exactly what transpired during the three decades of self-imposed *sadhana*. We only know that when he returned to the world of men he was a supremely enlightened sage. His first pilgrimage was through India, where he met Aurobindo, Sri Ramakrishna and others. From India, Govinda journeyed to Afghanistan and met the first Agha Khan, Hasan Ali Shah, and became well-acquainted with the Ismaili tradition. Then, he traveled on to Persia, to the Holy City of Mecca and to Jerusalem. All the while, he traveled on foot as he made his world pilgrimage, except for times a boat was necessary to cross the water. Eighty per cent of the land journey he made by foot, and it took him forty years, from 1875 to 1915, to circumambulate the planet. In most of the countries he visited, he was presented to the reigning sovereign.

After a visit to Rome, where he spent some time, he visited most of the countries of Europe. He met with Kaiser Wilhelm II and Queen Emma of the Netherlands. Govinda then spent four years in England and was a frequent visitor of the Queen. It is believed that he gave counsel to these persons of influence, but he would never discuss it in later years. During an encounter with George Bernard Shaw, he was told: "You Indian saints are the most useless of men; you have no respect for time." Govinda's reply was: "It is you who are slaves of time. I live in Eternity."

In America this great sage met with Theodore Roosevelt and spent two or three years here. Next came Mexico, South America, the Pacific Islands via New Zealand and Australia, Sinkiang and then Nepal. In Benares, he donated a large sum of money for the founding of the Benares Hindu University and was offered the Chancellorship, which he declined. After a final visit to his place of birth, he turned in the direction of Nepal and there settled in the Shivapuri Forest, leaving his former name behind forever. Thirty-eight more years were to be spent in quiet seclusion, a seclusion which was only broken on rare occasions, when he would receive spiritually aware seekers who were ready to take his clear message to heart.

To those who came for guidance, the Shivapuri Baba always stressed practical living, meditation and remembrance of God. His teaching was so simple that many found it subtle and even surprising. He emphasized what he referred to as Right Life, a life lived in accordance with nature. All of what he taught can be found in the *Bhagavad-Gita,* a text to which he frequently referred. The great beauty of this simple life is that it was the personification of the highest ideals of yogic tradition.

In his final talk with Mr. Bennett, he was asked for a summation of his teaching emphasis, and he said: "The sum and substance of my teaching is this: live the minimum life possible, subjecting body and mind to strict discipline. Again, how a very hungry man longs for meat, how a man suffering from intense cold longs for heat, so long for God, meditate on Him continously. And this is the sum and substance of my teaching. That is for you, that is for them, that is for the whole world. It is by this that I saw the Truth, and I am happy. Yes."

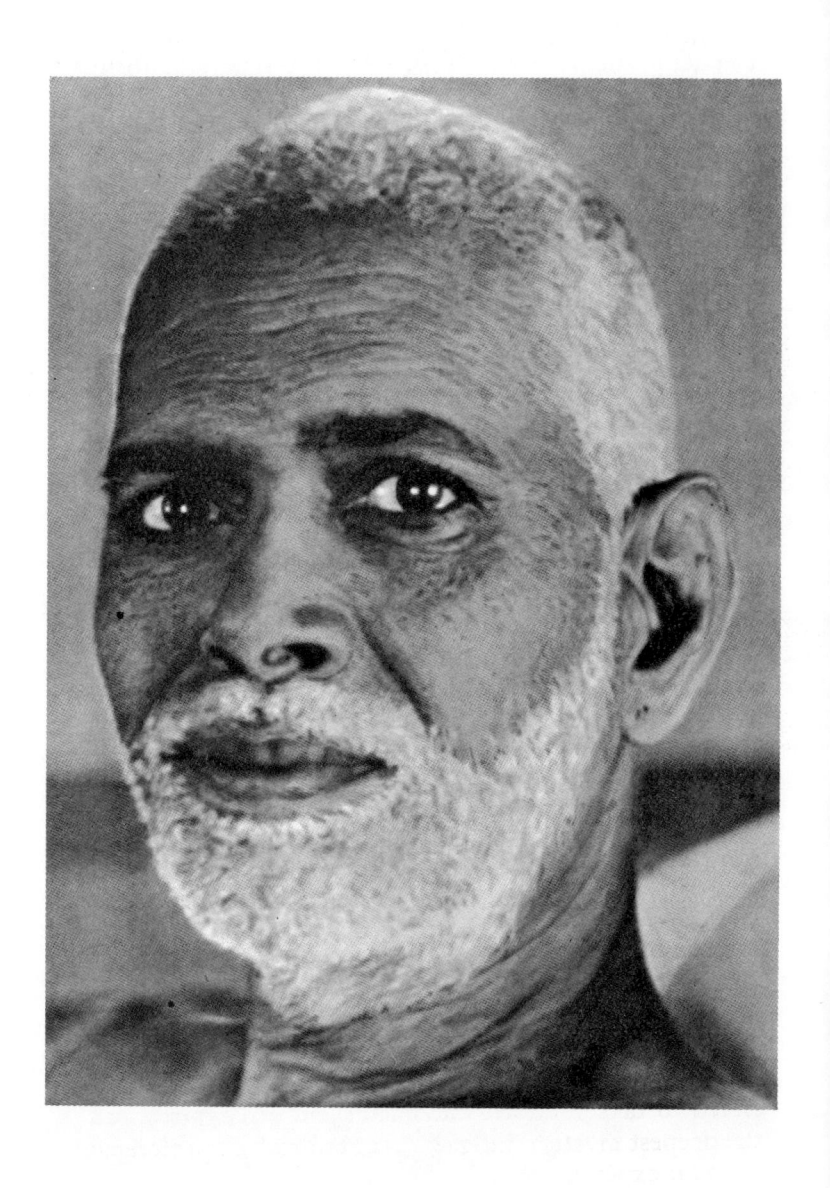

RAMANA MAHARISHI

Since the early part of the third decade of this century, many seekers found their way to a quiet man who lived in virtual seclusion in South India. At his ashram just below the majestic Arunachala, "the sacred red mountain," the illumined sage Ramana Maharishi remained anchored in the bliss of Self-Realization and served as a conduit through which the light of God found full expression.

There is little doubt but that Ramana Maharishi came into this world for a mighty purpose. As a young man with no prior religious training, he was suddenly stricken one day with a fear of death. His intelligence led him to examine the dying process. Thus he reclined and detached his awareness from the body, mind and feeling nature. He remained conscious and gained insight into the truth that his real nature was Witness Consciousness. Ever after he counseled seekers to practice Self-inquiry, to ask within, "Who am I?" until knowledge of the Self was clearly realized.

Before the Maharishi's realization was perfected, he was to undergo extreme inner cleansing experiences. It is one thing to have inner knowing, it is quite another to experience realization through body and mind without obstruction. After his initial insight, he went to a temple in South India, surrendered before the altar and asked God to consume him completely. What happened next is in line with the *Siddha* tradition; he experienced an immediate awakening of *kundalini*, which began to work spontaneously in him. For many months, the young devotee was led through all of the varied and complicated yogic processes. For days he was not inclined to take food. He remained silent and experienced the deepest mystical insights, as a result of his prolonged *samadhi* experiences.

As his inner purification continued, he sought seclusion in a cave on Arunachala, the mountain said to be the residing place of numerous *Siddha* adepts who dwell there in their subtle bodies. Even today it is said that lights can be seen moving about the mountain, and many believe these lights to be evidence of the *Siddhas*. Years after his public work began, Ramana himself declared this to be true.

This great sage was not destined to live out this incarnation in total seclusion for, in time, people began to regard him as a perfect master and came for his *darshan*. After a time, an ashram grew up around Ramana. He allowed it to grow but took no part in the management of ashram affairs. Paul Brunton met this master and wrote of him in his book, *A Search in Secret India*. The world beyond India's borders then began to know of Ramana Maharishi, and the pilgrims started to journey toward Arunachala.

Ramana Maharishi best exemplified the teaching emphasis of *Jnana Yoga*, because of his insistence upon using the faculty of intelligence to discern the truth about life and consciousness. He did not teach *pranayama* or any specific technique other than to inquire as to the Source of thought. When the mind is turned back upon itself, the masters teach, one flows the attention to the Source of mind which is Pure Consciousness.

While the sage seldom talked of *kundalini* experiences, his *shakti* was transmitted to receptive disciples, and they began to experience the spontaneous inner workings of the energy which has transforming power. The *shakti* flowing from the Maharishi also pervaded the ashram grounds, making it a true pilgrimage shrine, where seekers still come for the uplifting effect. While being an example of perfect knowledge, Ramana also was the personification of devotion, content to remain absorbed in Supreme Consciousness and letting God run the universe as He could best do it. One visitor asked, "How can we help the world?" The sage replied, "Mind your own business."

Though he never left his ashram environment, except for occasional walks along the mountain paths, his interest extended beyond the ashram and into the secular world. The Maharishi kept up with the news of world events through radio and newspapers, maintained an active correspondence with seekers and authored a few small books. His love extended to the animal kingdom, too, and the cows, dogs and other animals who lived there were given names and treated with full respect, even to the point of being given ritual burial when deceased.

When his aged mother was near death, the Maharishi sat with her for several hours, one hand over her heart and the other on her head. Through yogic attunement, he was able to know the contents of her subconscious mind and infused her with his own energy and intention. Thus, she worked out her karma through vivid vision, before resting in the clear state just prior to conscious transition. Such is the ability of a *Siddha* master.

Ramana Maharishi left his own body consciously in 1950, and a comet was seen streaking through the night sky at the moment of his departure. He was buried on the ashram grounds, and a shrine was erected over the body. Such a shrine is called a *samadhi*, because it is taught that here, where a master's body remains, his energy also remains. This energy charges the shrine with *shakti*, which others can receive if they meditate at the site with devotion and surrender to God.

Here is an example of the teaching of Ramana Maharishi: "Forgetting the Self, mistaking the body for It, going through innumerable births and finally knowing the Self, and being as the Self, is only like waking up from a dream of wandering all over the world."

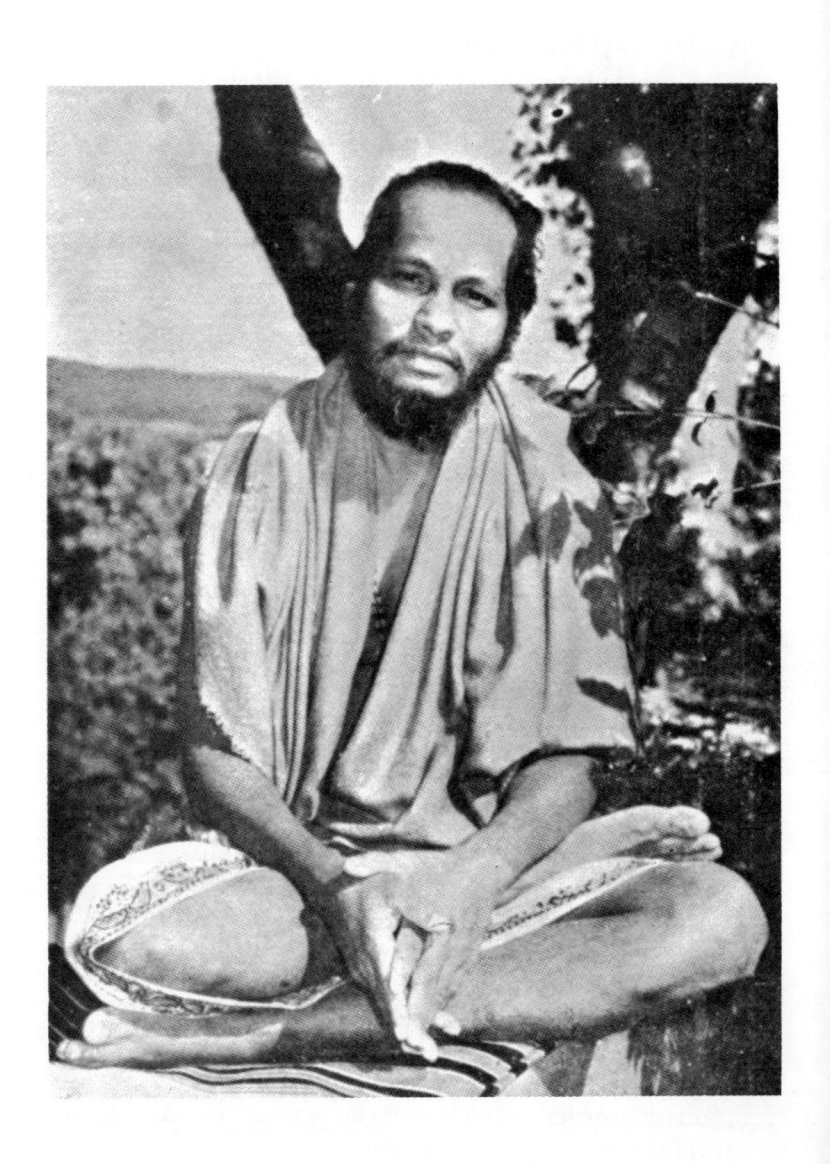

SWAMI MUKTANANDA PARAMAHANSA

"Bow to the Self within you, God dwells in you as you!" is the forthright statement frequently made by one of the authentic *Siddhas,* who has come into the world with the full impact of his *shakti* power. Swami Muktananda Paramahansa speaks with the conviction born of true God-Realization and awakens others to the Reality of God. His tradition is *Shaktipat Diksha,* initiation through awakening of the divine energy in others.

Swamiji was born May 16, 1908, at dawn. The place was Dharmasthala in Mysore State, a favorite pilgrimage site for thousands of devout persons. The child was named Krishna and, because his family was wealthy, they weighed him on a scale and gave a weight of gold and silver at the temple dedicated to Lord Manjunath. As a boy, he had a love of adventure and used to say often, "One day I will go to far, distant places of our country and learn many things."

The turning point in his life occurred when he was fifteen and met his future guru, the renowned Swami Nityananda. Revered as an *avadhoot,* a supremely enlightened renunciate and master of *Siddha* methods, Nityananda used to roam about South India and to shower his blessings on all who responded to his grace. The encounter was brief: Nityananda embraced Krishna and stroked his cheeks. Then he walked quickly away.

Six months later the teenage Krishna left home and went to Mysore. Here he was guided to the ashram of Siddharudha Swami, a great *Siddha.* At this ashram Krishna studied Sanskrit and the elements of Vedanta and Yoga. It was here that he was initiated into the monastic order and became known as Swami Muktananda.

For several years Swamiji traveled throughout India,

visiting shrines, ashrams and various holy men. It was at a place near Yeola, in the district of Nasik, that his most intense inner work was done. Here, in a hut provided by devotees who loved him, he experienced dramatic *kundalini* awakening, underwent months of inner transformation and experienced a variety of *samadhi* states. True to the inner leading of God, when the young yogi needed assistance, it appeared in the form of a true master in the *Siddha* tradition. He met Zipruanna, Harigiri Baba, Nrisinha Swami and Bapumai. Each master gave Muktananda specific help, but the crowning relationship was to be formed when Muktananda again met his guru, Nityananda, at Ganeshpuri, near Bombay.

Nityananda initiated his disciple and imparted the sacred mantra, *Om Namah Shivaya*, as the vehicle through which his blessing would be transmitted. Muktananda's *sadhana* became more intense as he practiced meditation for long hours daily. He later wrote concerning one of his early experiences: "I then saw blazes of fire on all sides and felt that I too was burning. Suddenly, a large ball of light approached me from the front; as it approached, it grew brighter and brighter. It came through the closed doors of my hut and merged into my head. My eyes were forcibly closed and I felt a fainting sensation. I was terrified by the powerfully dazzling light. I could see that light in my head. It would become bright, and then only darkness was perceived. Finally I saw a blue flame of light which grew larger, then diminished. Remaining steady, it was about the size of a small pearl, and it began to sparkle. Suddenly, my tongue became fixed in *khechari mudra* and I inwardly uttered the words 'Sri Gurudev' and everything became normal from that moment. All yogic *kriyas* ceased. The entire process had lasted over two hours."

Muktananda has written of his extraordinary experiences in his fascinating book, *Chitshakti Vilas* (*The Play of Consciousness*). Here, too, one learns of the beautiful relationship between Swamiji and his beloved guru, Nityananda. Several years before Muktananda's Enlighten-

Masters of Yoga

ment, Nityananda had settled at Ganeshpuri, which was once the site of an ancient temple of *Shiva*. A township grew up around the sage, and today there is also a large ashram which is Muktananda's world headquarters. Nityananda's *samadhi* shrine remains a pilgrimage site for thousands of persons who visit it annually. Sri Gurudev Ashram is one of the most beautiful ashrams in India, and this is a reflection of the devotion and the careful planning of Muktananda Paramahansa.

In 1970 Swamiji visited America. Thousands responded to his magnetism and *shakti* power. He returned in 1974 and established a large ashram in Oakland, California. Over twenty thousand disciples have attended his retreats, which have been offered in major regions of the country. He returned to India in the fall of 1976, joined by over three hundred disciples who made plans to continue their training with him at the ashram.

Muktananda's teaching process is to remind disciples of their innate divinity, to encourage them in the path of service and dedication to God, and to transmit his energy to those who are open to his grace. After this awakening, he teaches, spiritual progress is certain and steady.

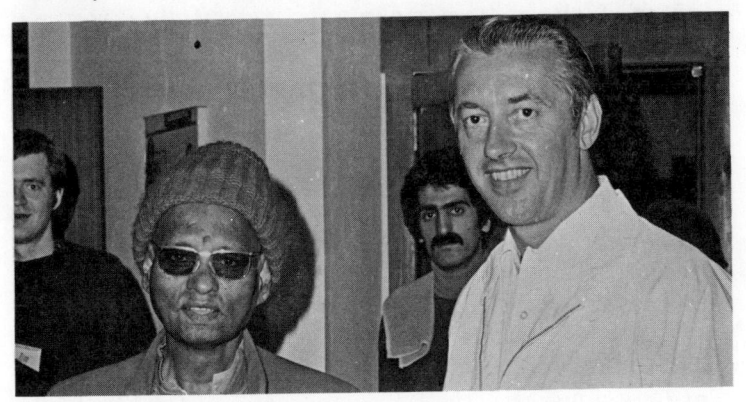

Swami Muktananda and the author in California. *Photo by Ron Lindahn.*

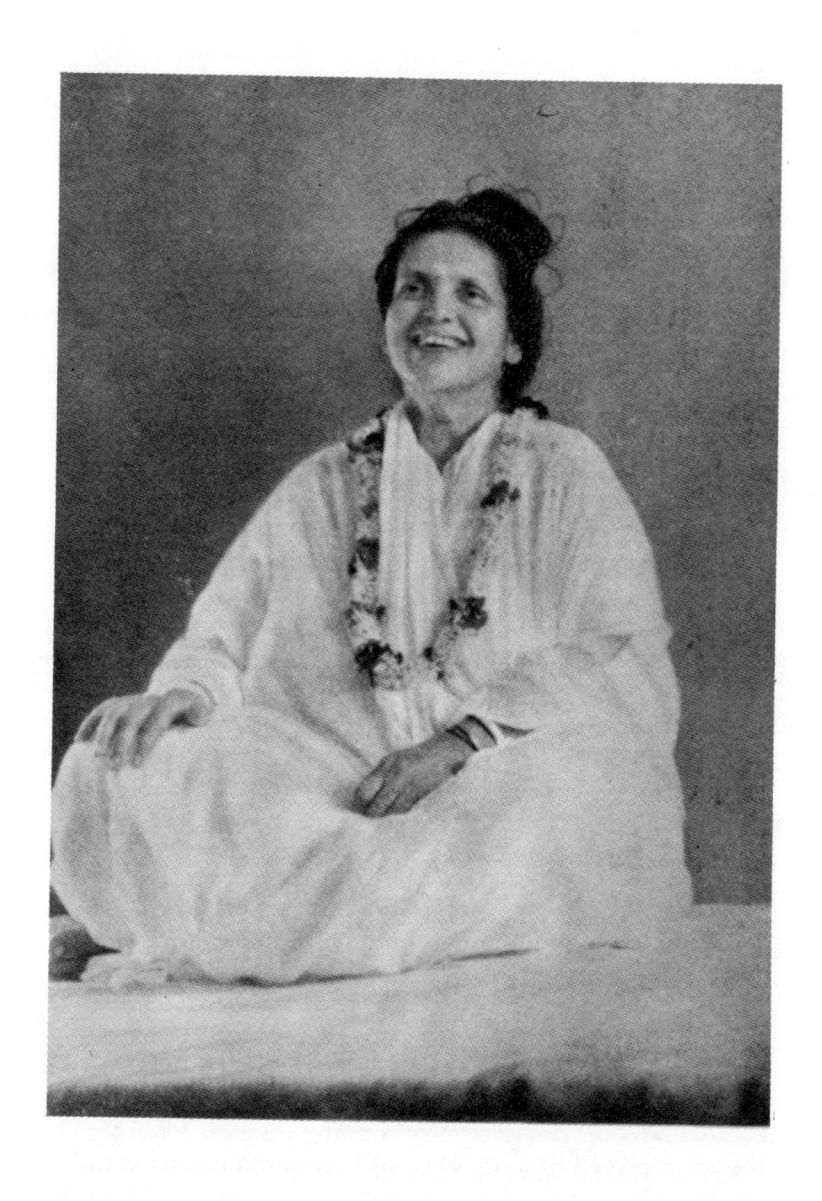

ANANDA MAYI MA

The life of Ananda Mayi Ma, the "Joy-Filled Mother," is another example of spontaneous awakening and a life of service. As a child, this great saint experienced all of the yogic processes without having ever been taught them in this incarnation. She has said that she came into this body with knowledge, and the early years were times of adjusting to her new form and her new environment.

When Paramahansa Yogananda talked with her in 1935, she shared with him the insight that she "lived in Eternity" and did not identify with the body, except for the purpose of remaining on earth to do God's will. She came into her body in May, 1896, at Tripura, a village in East Bengal. Her only formal schooling was two years of attendance at a lower primary educational institution.

Ananda Mayi Ma is revered by millions in India and is considered by many to be a Divine Incarnation. She not only teaches in the tradition of *Vedanta,* stressing the Reality of God and man's relationship to God, but encourages all to worship with devotion and to be true to their chosen way. As a means to control one's mental activity, Ma recommends *japa,* the repetition of God's name in whatever aspect the devotee most cherishes.

Over two dozen ashrams have been prepared for this saint, and she travels frequently from city to city, conducting *satsang* and leading devotional singing. Her personal counsel is avidly sought after by persons from all walks of life, and she treats everyone the same, as she sees only the One Life running through various forms.

No matter what her body is doing, Ananda Mayi Ma is ever centered in God. She has sometimes admitted to seeing people in their subtle forms who come for blessing, people who have left the body but are still attuned to the physical plane. She also recalls her previous incarnations and holds inner communion with other saints and sages, who live at a distance from where she happens to be. She was once asked how she saw her visions and perceived subtle realms. She responded: "How do I see them? Why, the eyes are all over the body. Don't you know that everything has in it the essence of all other things? Hands, legs, hair, in fact every part of the body can be made the instrument of sight. Of course, it is quite possible to see through the two eyes which we all possess, and the existence of a third eye of which you speak is also true. People do possess such eyes. This may sound strange to you, but nonetheless it is true."

In response to a question regarding the ability of a sage to assist others who suffer, she said: "Sages can mitigate the suffering of other people in three ways. They can take the suffering upon themselves and thus relieve the sufferer; they may distribute the karmic debt among others (who are willing to share the problem). It may also happen that sages, through their grace, can relieve an individual from all the consequences of his actions and restore him to Life Divine, which is the true Self."

Rarely does Ananda Mayi Ma talk about herself. Occasionally, when pressed by a devotee, she will share a little of her understanding. For instance, she once was asked about her ability to heal and to bless. Her reply was: "When *siddhis* (the powers of perfection) become one with the Supreme Self, then they are regulated by the Supreme Self. In this realization there is no room for the play of the limited personality. I have known this from infancy. Let me tell you that what I am, I have been from my infancy. But when the different stages of *sadhana* were being manifested through this body, there was something like a superimposition of *ajnana* (ignorance due to identification with nature). But this was really a case of knowledge masquerading as ignorance. Let me tell you a story relating to my childhood. Once a woman became pregnant in our village, and her child was born in due time. I knew from the beginning that the child would not live long. He had only come to complete his cycle of births and deaths. After a year he became ill, and I went to him and gave him my blessing by placing a hibiscus flower under his pillow. I did this under the urge of the Supreme Self. At the stage of *sadhana*, soul power first manifests itself as you, which may come, for instance, from the recitation of God's name. When people experience this, they may think that they have got everything that *sadhana* can yield, and their upward progress is thereby arrested. But he who keeps himself always on the move, without being overwhelmend by such manifestations of joy, finds himself in possession of various miraculous powers. But those powers are not meant for display. They should be carefully kept under control. He alone can know his true Self, who keeps alive within him an insatiable thirst for the Divine, without being contented with the possession of supernormal powers. Such powers may enable one to cure any disease by a mere touch of the hand or may lead to the fulfillment of one's desires."

In the tradition of the *Siddhas*, Ananda Mayi Ma not only offers herself as a living embodiment of the Divine, she also steadily exhorts her listeners to persist on the path. She says: "God is. Whatever you behold is nothing but a manifestation of Him. Once you know Him and live in Him, there is an end to all your sorrows and sufferings. You then realize supreme Bliss, eternal Joy. Strive hard, therefore, to realize Him. Remember, there is no peace without God. How are you to take that path? Be desperately eager; sincerely desire to find out. That will make your path easy. Pray to Him who is ever gracious: 'My Lord, I want you. Have mercy upon me.' Weep for God. If you have been initiated by a *Guru*, well and good. Remember, it is God who manifests Himself as the Guru. Even if you have not been initiated, do not cease to strive. Take refuge in Truth. At all times engage yourself in activities as would kindle within you a longing for God. Always try to see that He is everything and everyone, that all creatures are but manifestations of Him. No matter what you are doing, the underlying idea should be that by doing it you are only serving Him, fulfilling His purpose. Your son is nothing but God in the guise of a child. Who is your daughter? She is *Kumari*, the primeval *Shakti*. Your husband is a manifestation of the Lord of the universe. Your wife represents the goddess presiding over the household. Ideas of this kind should be cherished in the mind. Further, let truthfulness, renunciation, control of the senses and patience be always with you as your constant companions."

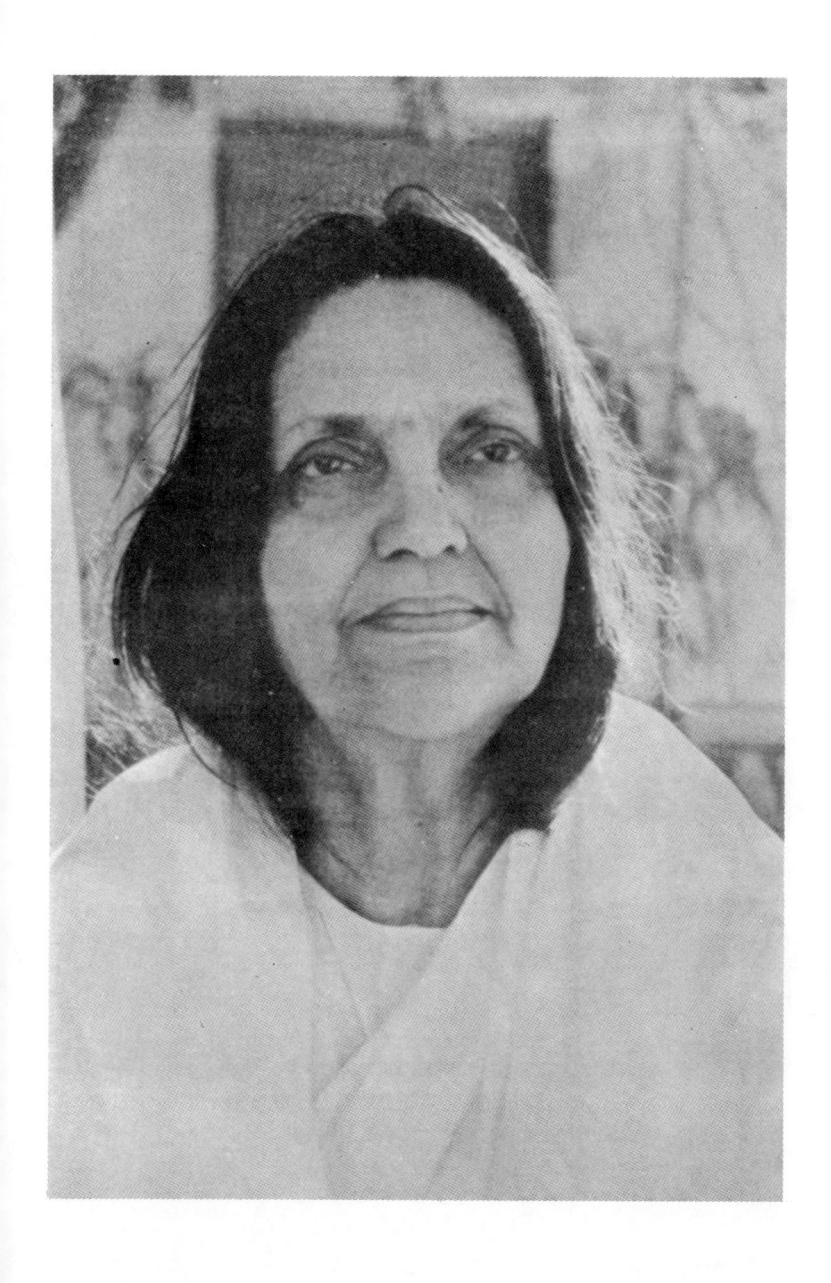

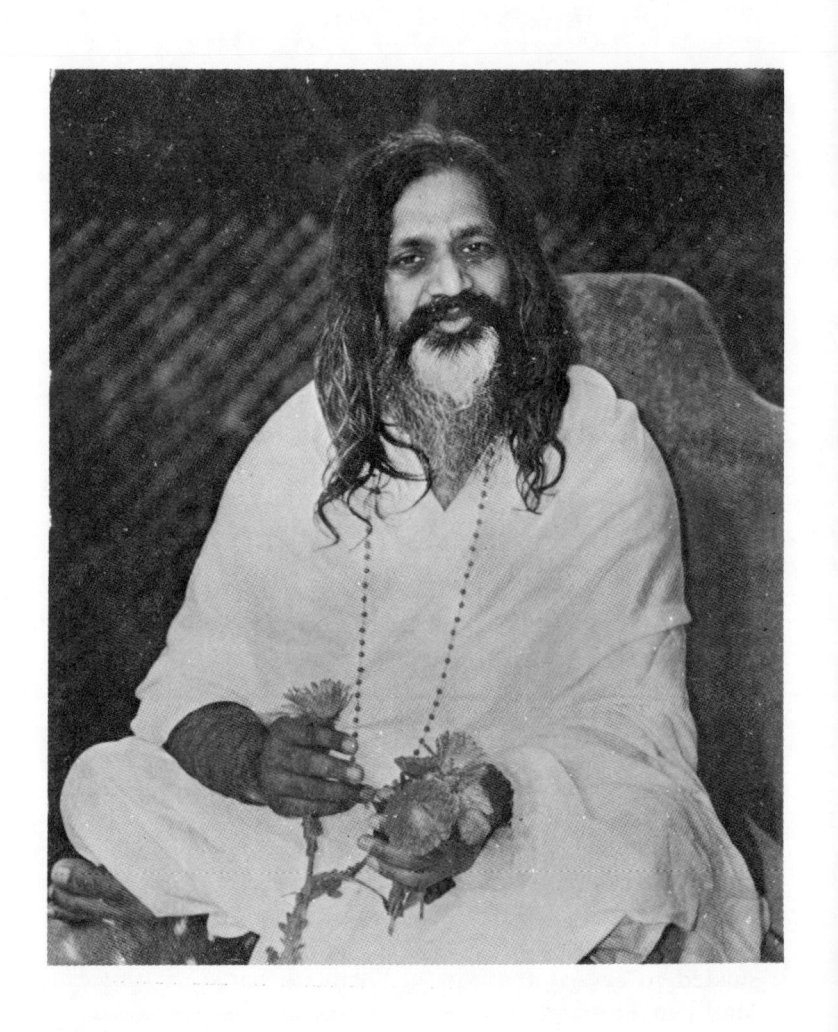

MAHARISHI MAHESH YOGI

When a man's message is very avidly accepted, with positive results following, the man must be an instrument of the Divine for the good of the world. Such a man is the one known to millions as Maharishi Mahesh Yogi, the moving genius behind the Transcendental Meditation Organizations.

Buckminster Fuller wrote: "What makes Maharishi beloved and understood is that he has manifest love. You could not meet with Maharishi without recognizing instantly his integrity. You look into his eyes and there it is."

Born Mahesh Prasad Varma in the central provinces of India, around 1918 (so one biographer has it), he was born into the caste of *Kshatriyas,* the warrior caste. His duty is to "defend the faith," to uphold the traditions of the *Vedas.* It is known that he graduated from Allahabad University in 1940, with a degree in physics. Before long he was to seek out his guru, the renowned Swami Brahmananda Saraswati, one of the four *Jagadgurus* (the world teachers among the Hindus, who are appointed to the post because of their intellectual qualities and superior God-Realization).

Swami Brahmananda had left his home while a youth to search for Enlightenment. He was initiated by his guru, Swami Krishnananda, and studied with him for many years, finally attaining full realization. For twenty-five years, Brahmanandaji remained in seclusion to perfect his yogic attainment. He was finally persuaded to accept the post of Shankaracharya of Jyotir Math, in Badarinath, the Himalayas, in 1941. As Shankaracharya he taught the meditation techniques originating in the *Vedas.* He was seventy-two years of age when Maharishi Mahesh Yogi came to him for instruction. For thirteen years, Maharishi served his guru and learned from him the ancient science of Soul-Realization. Even today, when he speaks, Maharishi has a large photograph of his guru behind him and tells people: "He expounded the Truth in its all-embracing nature. His quiet words, coming from the unboundedness of his heart, pierced the hearts of all who heard him and brought Enlightenment to the mind. His message was the message of the fullness of heart and mind."

For three years, after the passing of his guru, Maharishi remained in seclusion in Uttar Kashi, in the Himalayas. Under inner guidance, he left his retreat and journeyed to a town in the south of India. There, he met a man who invited him to speak to members of his community. The talks were so popular that the crowds grew daily, and Maharishi's public work began to gather momentum. In 1958 he felt the call to take his easy meditation system to the world, and a master plan was drawn up for this purpose.

Being in the tradition of the vedic seers, Maharishi obviously knows the scriptures and is well educated in yogic science. But, for mass teaching, he decided to emphasize a simple result-producing meditation method, that of listening to the internal sound. In this science of *mantra,* it is known that certain sounds have specific effects on the mind and the nervous system. Thus, *mantras* are given to initiates, according to the need of the individual.

Realizing that he could not possibly personally initiate ten per cent of the planet's population, which is his goal for improving the quality of society, he decided to train teachers who could take the science of meditation to the masses. So successful has this program been that by 1976 it was estimated that 600,000 Americans alone had been taught their personal *mantra.* TM meditators on a global scale must number well over one million, and the movement is accelerating in popularity.

Of course, what Maharishi is teaching is not a new method at all, but he has streamlined and simplified the presentation, so that almost anyone can derive practical results from the practice of meditation. Independent research has clearly indicated that correct meditation does reduce stress in the body, rest the involuntary nervous system, clear the mind and awaken energy in the system. One aspect of the TM teaching that draws occasional criticism is that of money being paid by initiates when they receive their *mantra*. This is entirely in accord with yogic tradition. The one who receives the benefit of the teaching has a responsibility to show appreciation, and the best way is often to support the organization which spreads the message.

From published reports, Maharishi lives a carefully disciplined life. While making full use of all modern communication tools, he seems untouched by ,the world. His food is simple vegetarian fare, his life is totally dedicated to world service, and once a year he secludes himself in his room for a week, taking with him only a small quantity of water. This is his occasion for recharging his system and preparing for the work ahead.

In 1975 a university was established in Iowa, and several hundred young students immediately enrolled. A full course is offered, featuring *Vedic* studies applied to the needs of today's world. This course is called *The Science of Creative Intelligence*. Hundreds of training centers provide instruction and meditation classes to seekers all over the world, retreats are offered for more in-depth work, and television stations are being planned to take the message to millions more.

Basically, Maharishi's intention is to inspire millions of persons to meditate and still to retain their active involvement with society. In this way, he teaches, as the quality of the mind and consciousness is enhanced, this improved quality will filter into the social consciousness and assist in the evolutionary process of mankind.

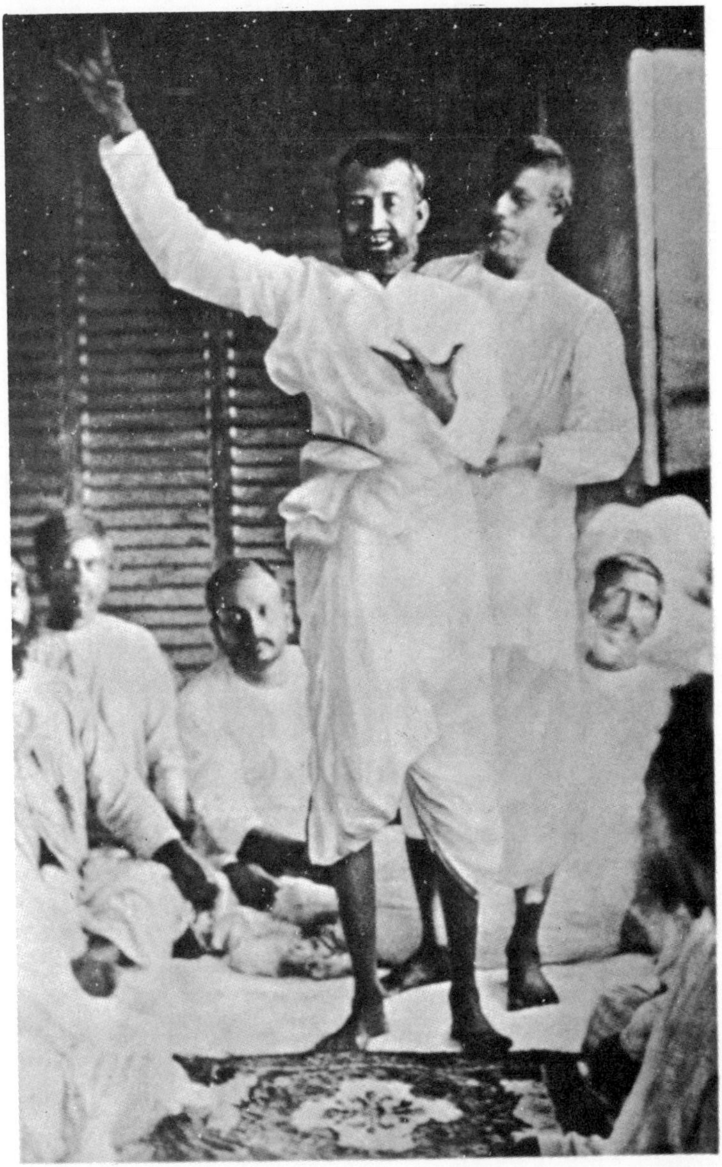

SRI RAMAKRISHNA PARAMAHANSA

In the final decades of the last century, a spiritual revival swept through Bengal, the western part of India. One of the most colorful saints in recent memory drew devotees of God to his side as nectar draws bees. Sri Ramakrishna was his name, and his spiritual influence has been felt around the world although he, himself, never made any efforts to preach or to write any books. His personal life and inspired teachings awakened souls and transformed lives.

In 1836, in the village of Kamarpukur, the soul who was later to be known as Sri Ramakrishna was born and named Gadadhar by his father. The name means "Bearer of the Mace" and is one of the epithets applied to God as *Vishnu*. A horoscope was drawn up for the child and indicated that he would live in a temple, surrounded by disciples; that he would found a new institution for teaching religion; and that he would be revered for generations to come. Interestingly enough, this information also confirmed the visions both parents had experienced prior to their son's birth.

Between the ages of six and seven, Gadadhar had his first intense religious experience. Later, his own words: "One morning I took some parched rice in a small basket and was eating it, while I walked along the narrow ridges of the rice fields. In one part of the sky, a beautiful black cloud appeared, heavy with rain. I was watching it and eating the rice. Very soon, the cloud covered almost the whole sky. And then a flock of cranes came flying by. They were as white as milk against that black cloud. It was so beautiful that I became absorbed in the sight. Then I lost consciousness of everything outward. I fell down, and the rice was scattered over the earth. Some people saw this and came and carried me home."

Though outer consciousness was absent, the boy reported that his inward awareness remained.

As he grew older, Gadadhar frequently fell into an ecstatic condition when thinking of God while at worship. Religious dramas would arouse his devotion and carry him into superconscious states. As a young man, he was invited to perform the worship (*puja*) in the *Kali* Temple at Dakshineswar. *Kali* is the aspect of God worshiped as *Shakti* Power, that which gives life and that which takes it away. In other words, the cosmic drama is considered to be the "play of Divine Mother" and can be understood as such. While at private prayer before the image of *Kali*, the young temple priest would pray: "Mother, you showed yourself to Ramprasad (a great devotional saint) and other devotees in the past. Why won't you show yourself (your real form) to me?" He would weep tears of despair and love.

In time a breakthrough came, and Ramakrishna began to experience long periods of ecstatic bliss, tremendous visions and powerful *kundalini* activity. As is common with great spiritual personages, when they show dramatic behavioral patterns which are considered "not quite normal" by their family members, Ramakrishna's family decided to arrange to have him marry. They hoped it would settle him down and have him attend to more responsible social matters. The marriage was arranged, but the result was that Ramakrishna's wife also had spiritual tendencies and, as the years passed, fully supported him in his quest. Years later, after Ramakrishna's passing, his wife became known as the Holy Mother and became a pillar of strength to disciples and devotees of the master.

We are informed by biographers that Ramakrishna studied the scriptures with various qualified teachers, mastered intricate Yoga practices and even practiced *tantric* rites with a woman initiate of this particular ritual. The last major contact came when he met his guru, Tota Puri, a member of a sect of yogis who went about naked. Tota Puri was an exponent of non-dualism, total identification with Supreme Consciousness without relative appearances. Even though he was married, Ramakrishna took the vows of a renunciate and accepted intiation from his guru. When he sat to meditate, after his instruction and initiation, the vision of Divine Mother flooded his mind. Ramakrishna explained: "As soon as Mother's form appeared, I took my knowledge of non-duality as if it was a sword in my hand, and I cut Mother (the vision) in two pieces with the sword of knowledge. As soon as I'd done that, there was nothing relative left in the mind. It entered the place where there is no second—only the One."

This was Ramakrishna's first experience in *nirvikalpa samadhi*, the Realization of Pure Being, with no concept or perception of anything other than *being*. Eleven months after he had arrived at Dakshineswar, Tota Puri was satisfied that his disciple was firmly established in God, so he left and never returned.

It was Ramakrishna's desire to remain permanently in the highest *samadhi*, but his inner guidance informed him that he had a mission in the world, and it would be best for him to remain at the level of *bhavamukha*, cosmic consciousness while embodied. In this manner he was able to continue to teach and to serve devotees who began to flock to him.

Toward the end of his life, he yearned for "true disciples," who would be able to comprehend him fully and to receive his *shakti* and take it to the world. Gradually, his helper-disciples came: Swami Vivekananda is best known to the public, but there were others. A few are Brahmananda, Shivananda, Turiyananda, Premananda and Saradananda. Vivekananda was the one chosen to take his master's message and the message of *Vedanta* to the western world, and he did it with enthusiasm and hard work of heroic proportions. Several *Vedanta Centers* in Europe and America today are directly the result of Vivekananda's pioneer efforts.

Ramakrishna told some of his disciples that Vivekananda had agreed, before taking birth, to come to the earth plane to assist him. The master said that when the disciple's work was finished, he would awaken to the realization of his real nature and leave his body. This is exactly what happened.

One of Ramakrishna's close disciples, Mahendranath Gupta, took notes whenever he was around the master. Later he produced a monumental book, *The Gospel of Sri Ramakrishan,* which gives insight and information seldom made available to the public, regarding the lifestyle and the teaching of a saint whom many consider to be an Incarnation of God.

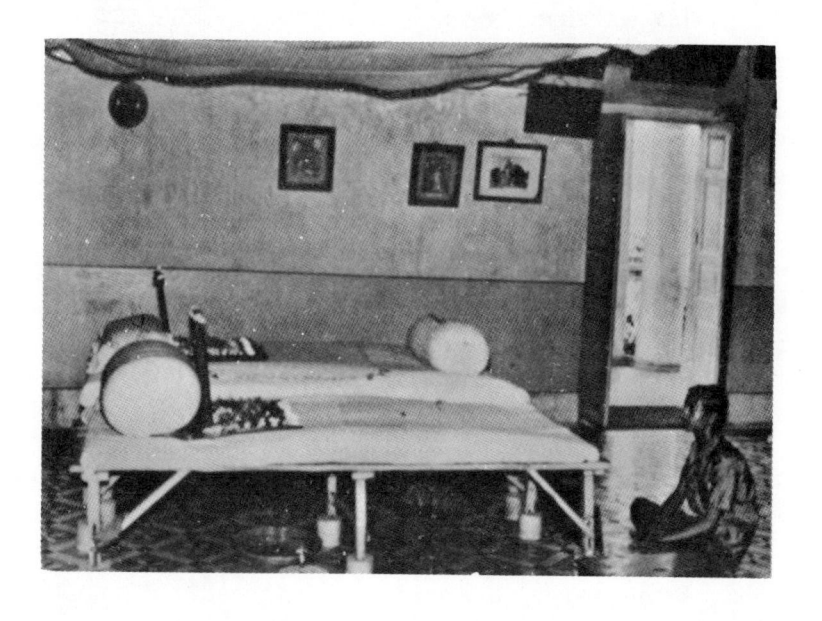

Ramakrishna's room at Dakshineswar

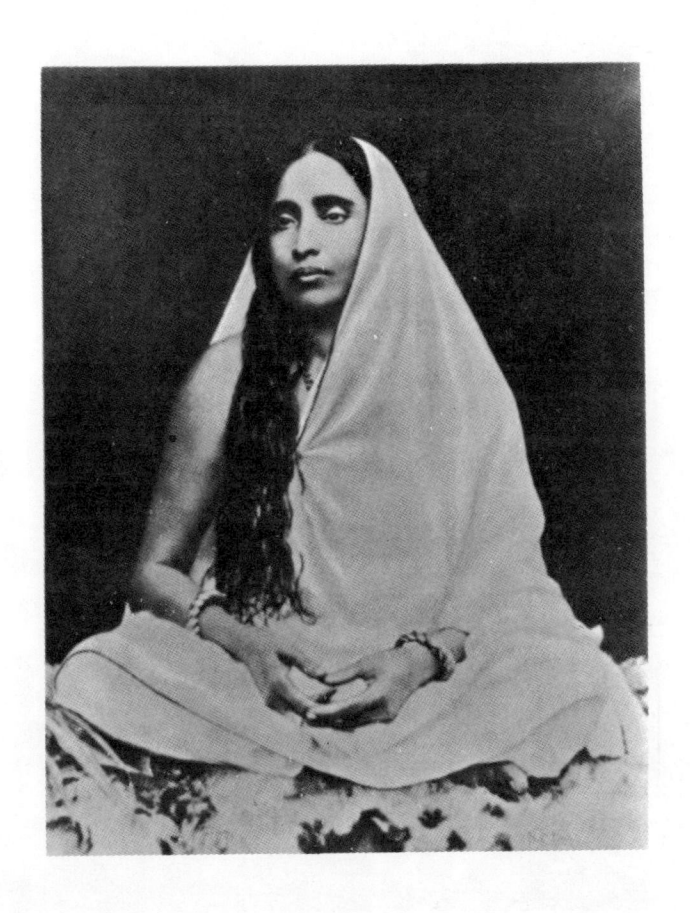

Sarada Devi, the Holy Mother

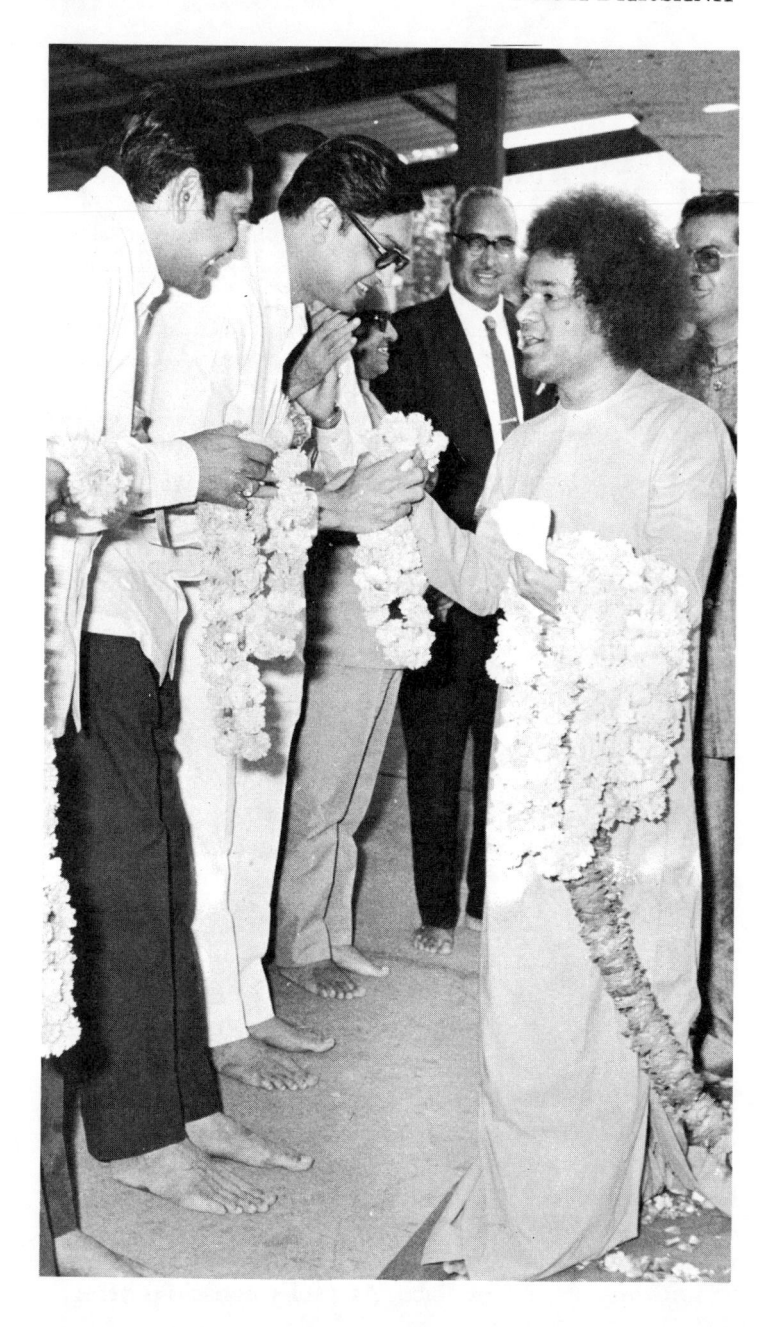

SRI SATYA SAI BABA

In southern India, one hundred and twenty miles northeast of the city of Bangalore, is the home of a holy man known as Sri Satya Sai Baba. Through him high inspiration flows and genuine miracles (*siddhis*) are manifested daily. At least one million devoted seekers visit his ashram, Prasanti Nilayam, each year, and additional millions are touched in person when he tours the country to give his message and his blessing. He gives of himself, for, as he says, "My life is my message."

Satya Sai Baba's realization is not the result of *sadhana* performed in this incarnation. He was born with all of the soul powers and came with a mission. This holy man does have close disciples, but he does not publicly speak of being a *guru*. He has chosen, instead, to work with the masses and to inspire them to awaken for the good of India and the world.

Born in the small village of Putta Parthi on November 23, 1926, Baba's fame has spread around the world. His ashram is just a few hundred yards from the village of his birth. He was born at the place where his future headquarters were to be. Millions of persons consider Sai Baba to be an *avatara*, an Incarnation of God. This means he is considered to be one who has consciously taken birth not for his own enlightenment experience, but born with knowledge and power for the good of others.

Satya Sai Baba recalls his previous incarnation as the beloved Shirdi Sai Baba, whose large ashram in the village of Shirdi is today a shrine and designated as such by the Indian Government. The holy man has said he will be in his present body until he is in his ninth decade, and then he will leave it. Shortly after that time, he will return in a new body in another part of South India and be known as Prema Sai Baba. As a fully conscious being, he knows his past experiences, his present duties and his future destiny.

At the age of fourteen, Satya left school to begin his work of teaching all who would come. His name spread throughout India and, before long, nearby property was acquired for the purpose of building an ashram. Prasanti Nilayam ("the abode of peace") is more a pilgrimage site than an ashram. There is little specific training offered, and most who come do so to see Sai Baba and to receive instruction and blessings. One of the more unique aspects of Baba's work is that he freely and spontaneously performs miracles. Since he is established in God, he has no egotistical need to impress anyone; he does what he does to meet human needs and to inspire faith. Almost everyone who has been with him for a short time has seen him stir the air with his hand and produce any number of articles: holy ash, prayer beads, rings, photos of saints and even medicine for one who might be ill. He possesses all of the *siddhis*, and they are expressed through him easily and without any evidence of effort on his part.

Another unusual aspect of his work is that he encourages his followers to take an active role in the community and even to build colleges for the education of India's youth. A feature of his educational system is that students are taught to understand the religions of the world and to embody the traditions of the *Vedas*. They are also taught devotional singing, meditation and the importance of service to humanity. Over three thousand centers and study groups throughout India and the world offer classes and devotional services.

As far as Sai Baba's teaching goes, it is in the tradition of the masters. Emphasis is placed on the remembrance of God at all times, daily worship, seeing others as divine and rendering service with a cheerful attitude. He does not teach specific methods or techniques but will often privately give *mantra* instruction and other advice as individual needs are observed.

There are recorded instances of Sai Baba's spiritual

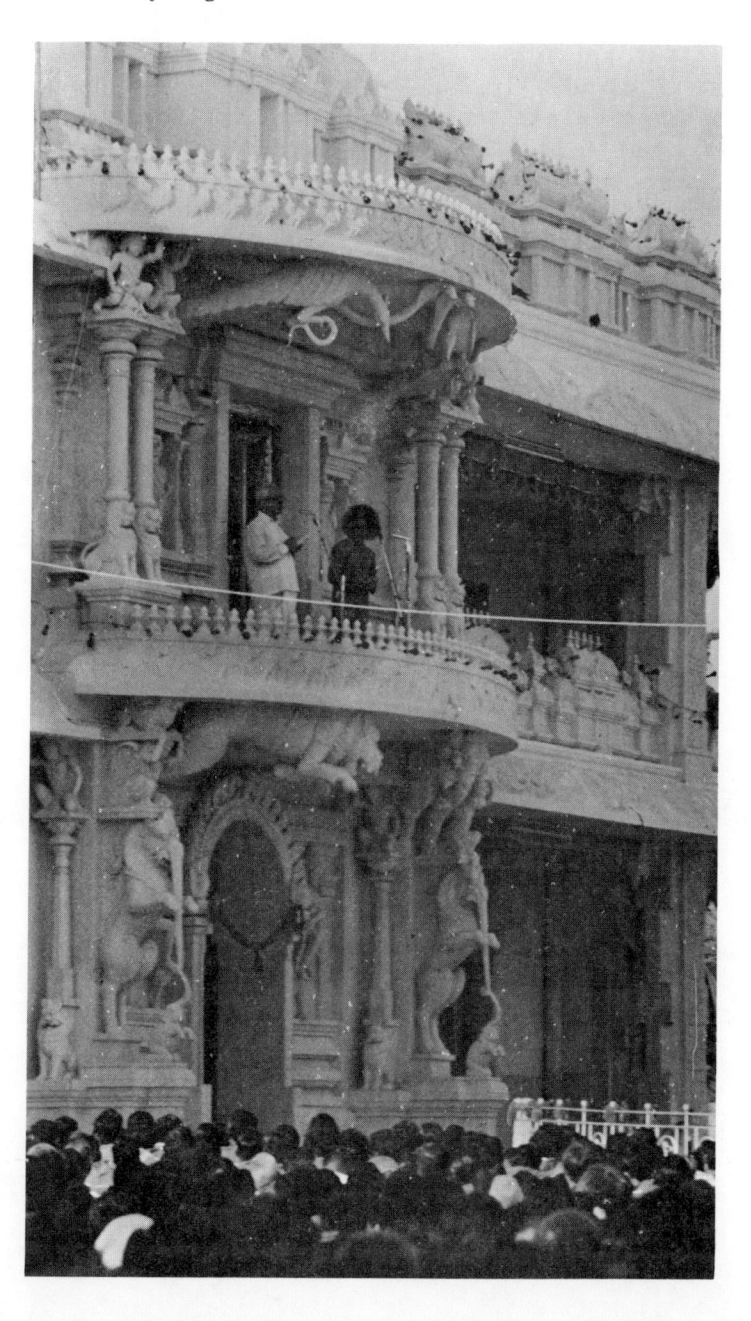

help in time of need, even when he is hundreds or thousands of miles from the one he is helping on the inner planes. He has also brought back life into bodies thought to be dead when the person being helped has karmic needs yet to be fulfilled. Even in India this holy man is a controversial figure because of his spontaneous methods and easy production of miracles. To him, however, what he does is simple, because he works from the level where he clearly understands the nature of Consciousness *as* the world.

It is very rare for a *Siddha* master to work so openly in public as Satya Sai Baba does. There have been others, of course, but this holy man is fully involved on such a large scale, because he feels that the world now needs such an influence. This is a time of global crises, as we move strongly into the new cycle before us. Such occasions require a powerful infusion of spiritual energy, so that the masses of people can be quickened and world consciousness cleansed for the work ahead.

"I have come," Sai Baba says, "to restore the world to the way of righteousnesss (*dharma*) and to remind people that no matter what their mode of worship, there is only one God and one humanity. My religion is the religion of love."

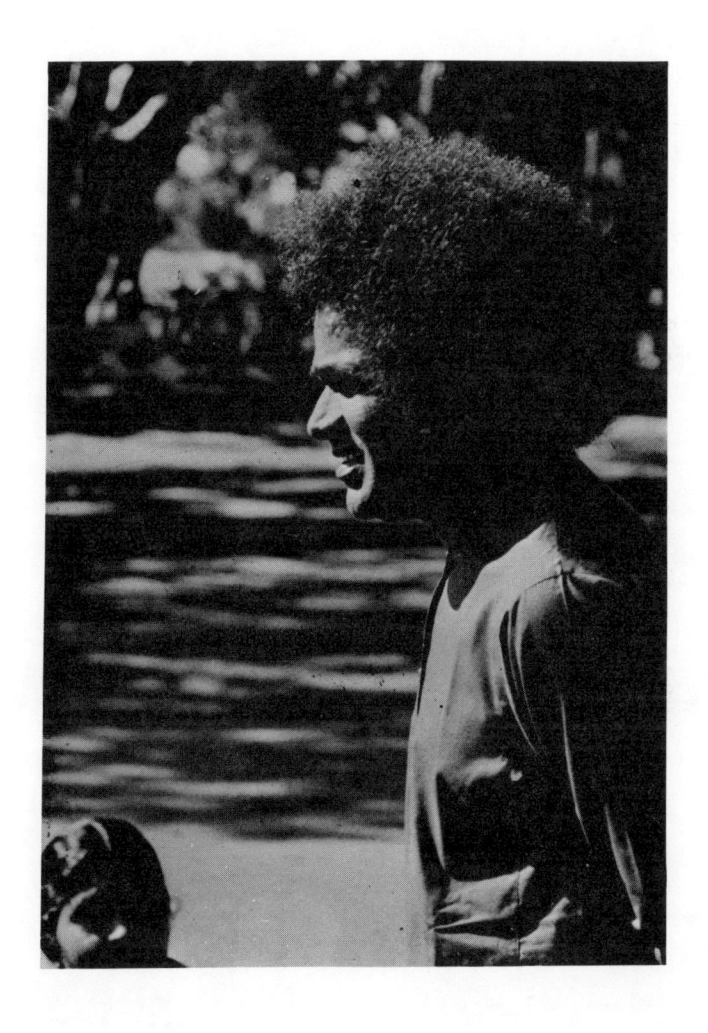

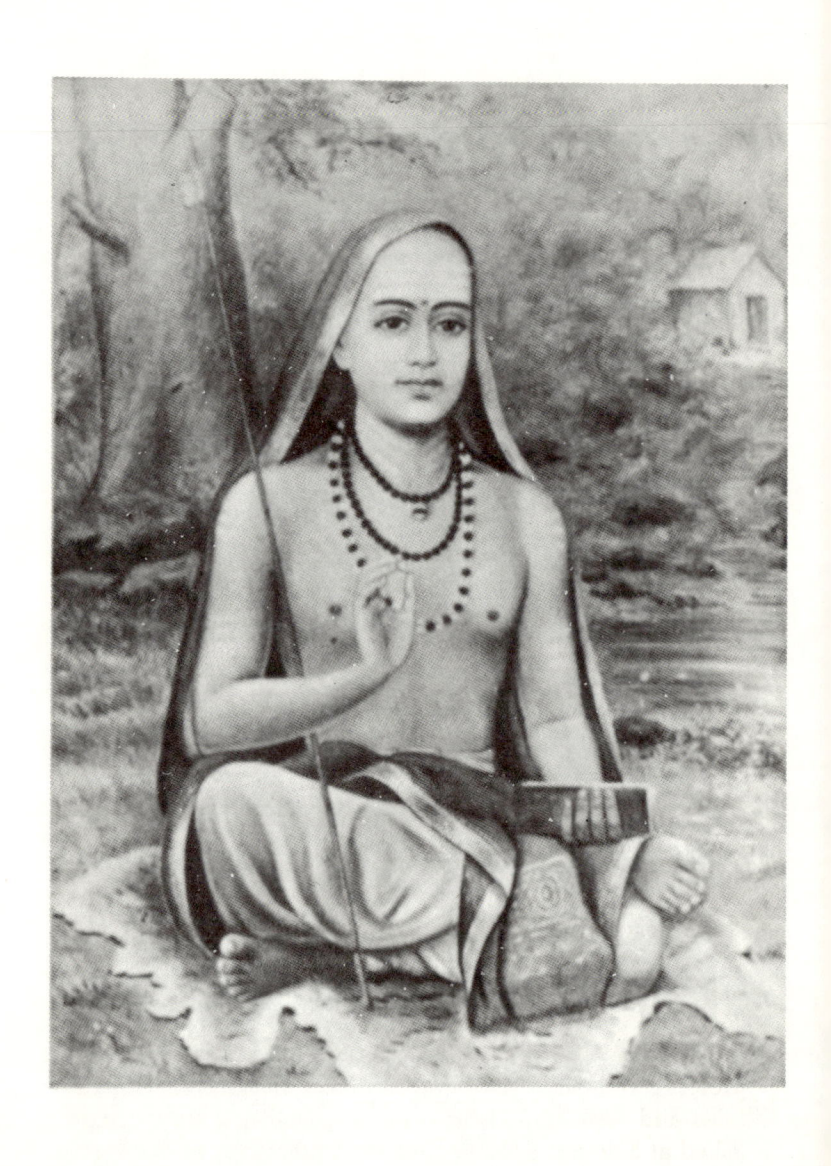

SHANKARACHARYA

Every swami belongs to the monastic order reorganized by *Adi*, (the first) Shankaracharya, who is revered even today as one of the great philosophical genius-seers of India. Shankara, as the name is sometimes used, not only revitalized the *Vedic* traditions and wrote extensive commentaries on the traditional texts, he also established four great centers of learning in the quarters of India, which today are seats of spiritual authority. Each of these four teaching centers is headed by a highly qualified leader who represents the unbroken spiritual tradition first established by the original Shankara. Each is known as the Shankaracharya (*acharya* means "teacher-sage") of the respective headquarters.

It is believed that Shankara lived in the eighth century after Christ and was born in the village of Kaladi on the west coast of South India. He mastered the scriptures at an early age and was initiated into the monastic life by the great ascetic Govindapada. He then devoted himself fully to *sadhana,* meditation and yogic practices. Because of his high realization and mastery of the scriptures, he was soon recognized as one of the lights of his time. Shankara felt the need to infuse new life into the religious practices of the people. To this end, he encouraged worship, study of the scriptures and a clear understanding of the message of the great sages. He traveled throughout India, meeting learned scholars in public debate as one way of bringing out the truths of the *Vedas.*

The four monasteries he founded were designed to preserve the pure teaching emphasis he stressed in his talks and writings. These centers of learning were established at Sringeri (*Mysore*) in the south, Puri in the east, Dwaraka in the west and in the Himalayas in the north. In 1958, Self-Realization Fellowship sponsored a three-month's visit to America for the existing Shankaracharya of Puri, the venerable Bharati Krishna Tirtha. This was the first time in history that a Shankaracharya had traveled to the West, and he was received enthusiastically at leading universities and at public gatherings which were arranged for his talks.

Adi Shankaracharya is best remembered today for his priceless commentaries on the *Bhagavad-Gita,* the *Brahma-Sutras* and the principle *Upanishads.* One of his classic expositions is *Atma-Bodha* or *Self-Knowledge,* in which he set forth a treatise on *Advaita Vedanta,* the philosophy of non-dualism. The essence of Vedanta is *Tat Twam Asi* ("That Art Thou"). That refers to Supreme Consciousness, and everything perceived is Supreme Consciousness appearing-as. Nothing has reality of its own; the world is merely a play of lights and shadows, an extension of Consciousness.

There are conflicting opinions regarding his departure from the world scene. He was last observed at Kedarnath, in the Himalayas. Some are of the opinion that he left his body there, since his earth mission was accomplished. Others are of the opinion that he withdrew from identification with the body and subtle sheaths, and still remains in the Himalayas as a mortal-immortal, like Babaji and others.

In his commentary on *Self-Knowledge* Shankara wrote: "I am composing this treatise to serve the needs of those who have been purified through the practice of spiritual disciplines, who are peaceful in heart, free from selfish cravings and desirous of liberation." This famous collection of verses on the reality of life contains only sixty-eight brief and challenging statements. The final one is this: "He who, renouncing all activities, worships in the sacred and stainless shrine of Supreme Consciousness, which is independent of time, space and distance; which is present everywhere; which is the destroyer of heat and cold and the other opposites; and which is the giver of eternal happiness, becomes all-knowing and all-pervading and attains immortality."

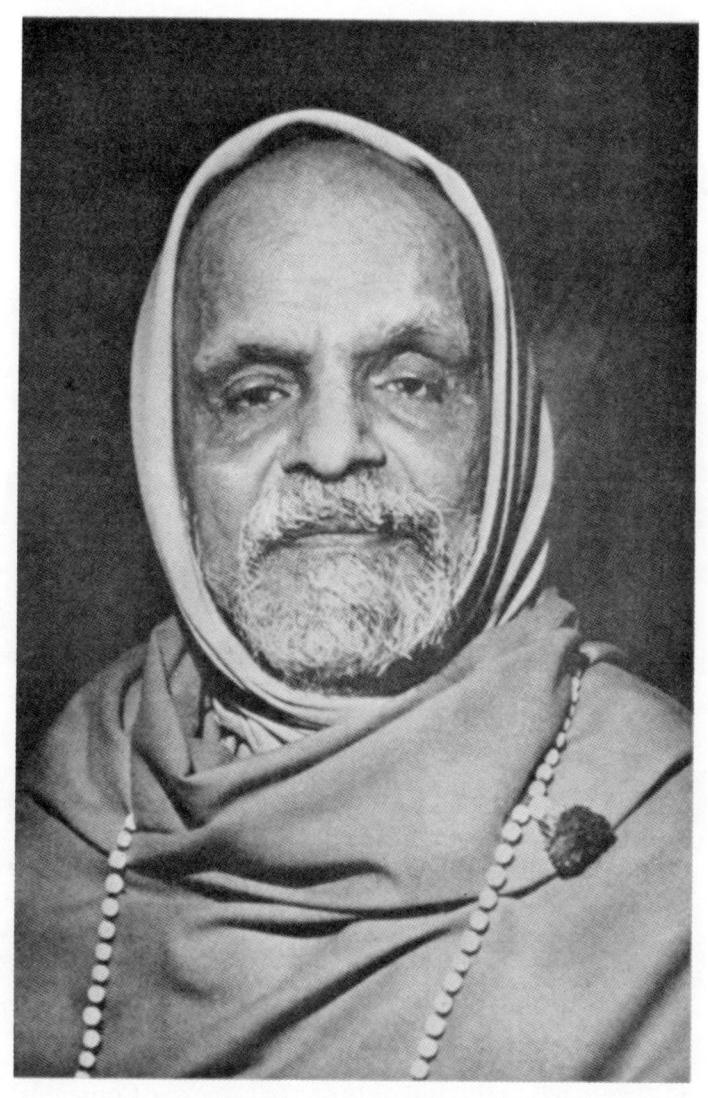

Shankaracharya Bharati Krishna Tirtha
1876-1961

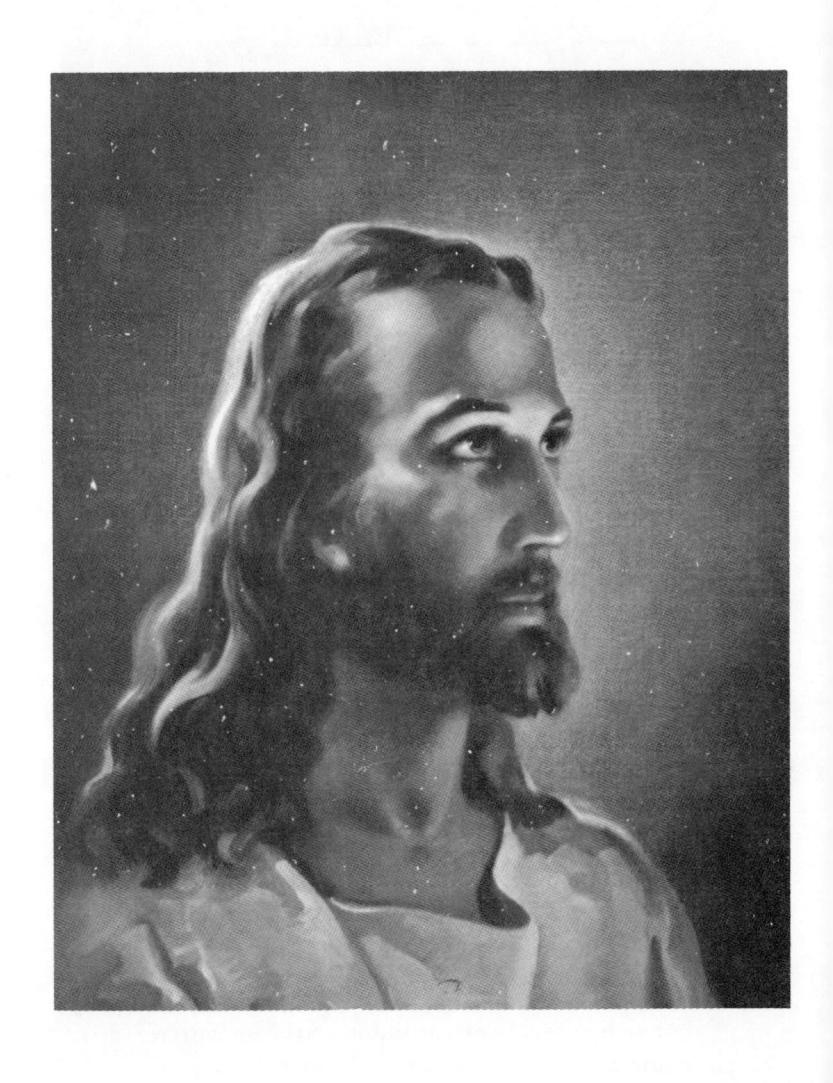

JESUS THE CHRIST

While not of the *Vedic* tradition, so far as we know, the example of Jesus, who was anointed with Christ Consciousness, must be taken as a manifestation of God in human form. Little of historical fact is known of Jesus, but the influence of his life upon multiplied millions of persons attests to his pure realization.

From *The Gospel According to St. John* and others, we clearly see the fairly common pattern of the work of a *Siddha* master who comes for a dramatic purpose. Supernatural happenings were common in the life of Jesus, indicating that he was an instrument of higher forces. We are told of the miracle of his birth, a usual occurrence for a world teacher, and of his knowledge and charisma as a child when he taught those older than himself. We find him seeking initiation at the hands of John the Baptist, experiencing an awakening, and then seeking out a quiet place for inner contemplation before beginning his public ministry.

True to the *Siddha* tradition, his first message to the people was: "Repent, for the Kingdom of Heaven is at hand." Every great master has taught the immediate availability of the heavenly state of consciousness as a result of one's returning consciously to an awareness of the Source. Jesus not only taught the way of inward turning and the importance of "praying without ceasing," he also moved freely among the people and showed partiality to none except, perhaps, those special ones who were pure in heart. He taught that the spiritual bond was more important than the physical and that one could overcome the world by coming into a close and a conscious relationship with God.

His miracles are also recorded: turning water into wine, materializing food for the multitudes, healing the sick, raising the dead and transforming lives with a word or a touch. Some see Jesus as a reformer, a teacher, an *avatara*, or even as simply a good man. We see him as a *Siddha* master, who went about doing only the will of God. He said: "I of myself can do nothing. The Father within, He doeth the works."

Jesus had disciples, and he chose them almost immediately upon meeting them for the first time. He knew who was called to assist him with his mission and the disciples responded, because of karmic ties and a destiny of world service. Some believe that John the Baptist and Jesus were, respectively, Elijah and Elisha of *Old Testament* fame. Elisha was a Hebrew prophet who succeeded Elijah as the leader of his people, and, in the *New Testament* story, Jesus went to John the Baptist to receive initiation. Jesus taught his disciples in private and transmitted his *shakti* power to them, so that they were able to teach boldly and to spread the message— the *good news* that man could awaken and become aware of his personal relationship with God and his fellowman.

The disciples of Jesus were admonished to love one another with the same love as they loved their *guru*. They were advised to follow the commandments or guidelines and to be examples to the world. They were taught to pray, not selfishly, but selflessly. Before his departure, Jesus brought his disciples together in a closed room and gave them final instruction in the mysteries. After his transition, he remained, in the tradition of many *Siddha* masters, in his subtle form and often appeared to disciples in their hour of need. He also worked through them after they had gone forth to teach in his spirit.

As is true with many masters, the teaching of Jesus has been widely interpreted, and many sects have been formed to teach a humanly accepted view of what he really meant to be given to the world. This matters little. The outer teaching serves the many, and the inner teaching, which is intuitively discerned, is always available to those who have eyes to see. Jesus taught the importance of initiation and stressed that the heavenly condition could not be known, unless one was "born again" or awakened from material consciousness to divine consciousness.

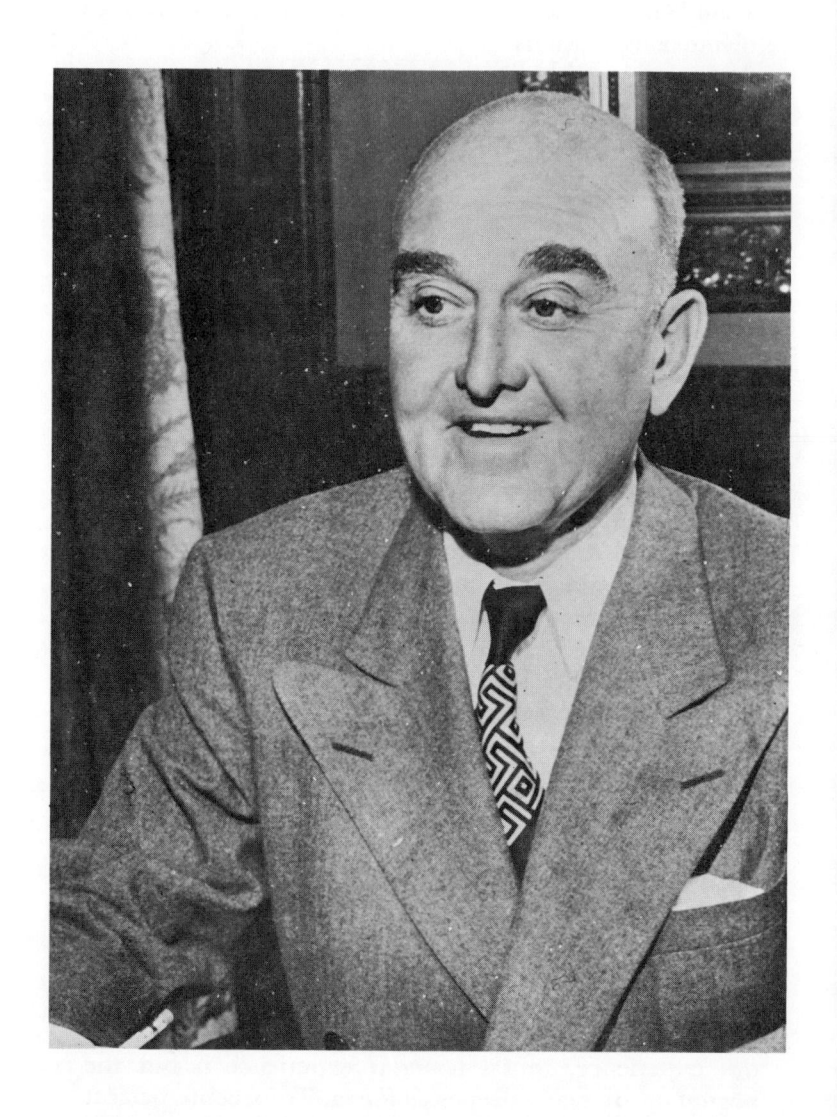

RAJARSI JANAKANANDA

In the summer of 1951, Paramahansa Yogananda publicly proclaimed an American businessman as his choice for the leadership of his organization. The monastic name given to his chosen disciple was Rajarsi Janakananda—and for good reason. Janak was a king and a saint in past ages in India. The disciple was also a combination of secular professionalism and spiritual insight. His name was James J. Lynn, and the midwest business community knew him as a multimillionaire businessman-philanthropist who headed a large oil interest and several insurance companies.

Mr. Lynn was already wealthy when he first met his *guru* in 1932, having worked his way through law school and becoming a certified public accountant, then moving up in the business world because of his brilliance and driving energy. He was later to say, "I had everything the world could offer, yet something was missing." Soon after his initiation into *Kriya Yoga*, the disciple experienced the first of several ecstatic states, which were a prelude to his final goal of *samadhi*. Yoganandaji told me of how he transmitted the *samadhi* experience to Mr. Lynn: "We were meditating one day by the ocean and I saw that he was ready. I touched him on the chest and he went into *samadhi*. He was oblivious of anything external and I watched him carefully."

For over two decades Mr. Lynn divided his time between Kansas City business responsibilities and California, where he spent most of his time in retreat for the purpose of enjoying the silence and deepening his *samadhi* experience. Initial *samadhi* experience is but the beginning of one's deeper *sadhana*. To become perfect in Yoga, one must continue to explore the more subtle aspects of mind and consciousness in order to burn out latent tendencies and to rest permanently in the exalted state.

Yoganandaji told many of us that Mr. Lynn (he called him "Saint Lynn") was a yogi in previous births and would attain final liberation in his present body. The two divine companions would spend hours in rapt meditation whenever possible. During one such meditation, they both saw a shaft of light descend upon them and remain for a time. Not only did Yoganandaji transmit his energy into his disciple, but Mr. Lynn also would frequently bless others and pass the current on to those who were receptive to it. I have told of this in my book *Darshan: The Vision of Light*.

While attending to his business duties, this great yogi adhered to a program of intense *sadhana*. It was his custom to awaken early in the morning, practice *asanas*, *pranayamas* and *mudras* and dive deep into meditation. He said: "The more I practice *Kriya Yoga* and the more I love God and Gurus, the more joyous and blissful I feel. I see that Master was right when he said, 'God is ever new.' "

Mr. Lynn was a strict vegetarian and, in later years, supervised the growing of organic foods on his farm in southern California, where he spent the final months of his life in meditation and close attunement with nature. Few of his business associates knew of his involvement in *Yoga*. Not until after his transition did the public become acquainted with the fact that he was a dynamic yogi, when the *Kansas City Star* carried a series of front-page articles detailing his life.

Retiring from business responsibilities shortly after Yoganandaji's *mahasamadhi* in 1952, Mr. Lynn spent more and more time in California, where he was an inspiration to his brother and sister disciples. Before his own transition, he arranged for several million dollars to be transferred from his estate to the organization founded by his *guru*.

All who remember him well recall his radiant nature and the strong *shakti* power that flowed from him. One visitor from India, after meeting Mr. Lynn for the first time, said: "Even in my native land, home of saints and sages, never have I been privileged to meet one such as him!" When he blessed others, Mr. Lynn would quietly whisper, "Master is blessing you, through me." As Yoganandaji often told us: "I am so pleased with Saint Lynn. He represents the best of both Western and Eastern principles. He has fulfilled all of my expectations for him."

A beautiful characteristic of this man's life is that he set an example for all who live in a world where responsibilities must be met, and he demonstrated that it is truly possible to fulfill practical obligations as well as to know God.

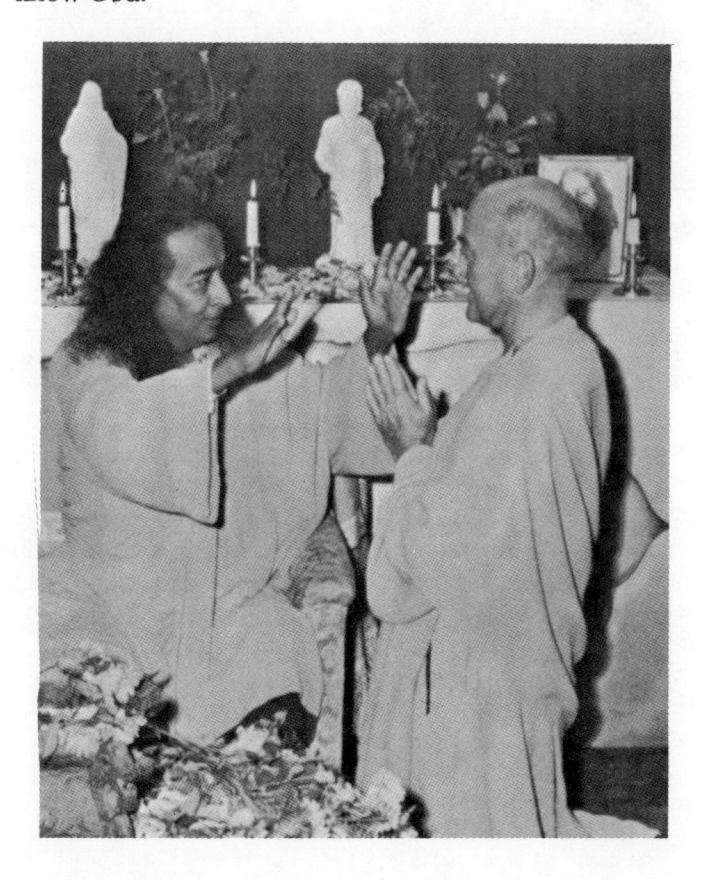

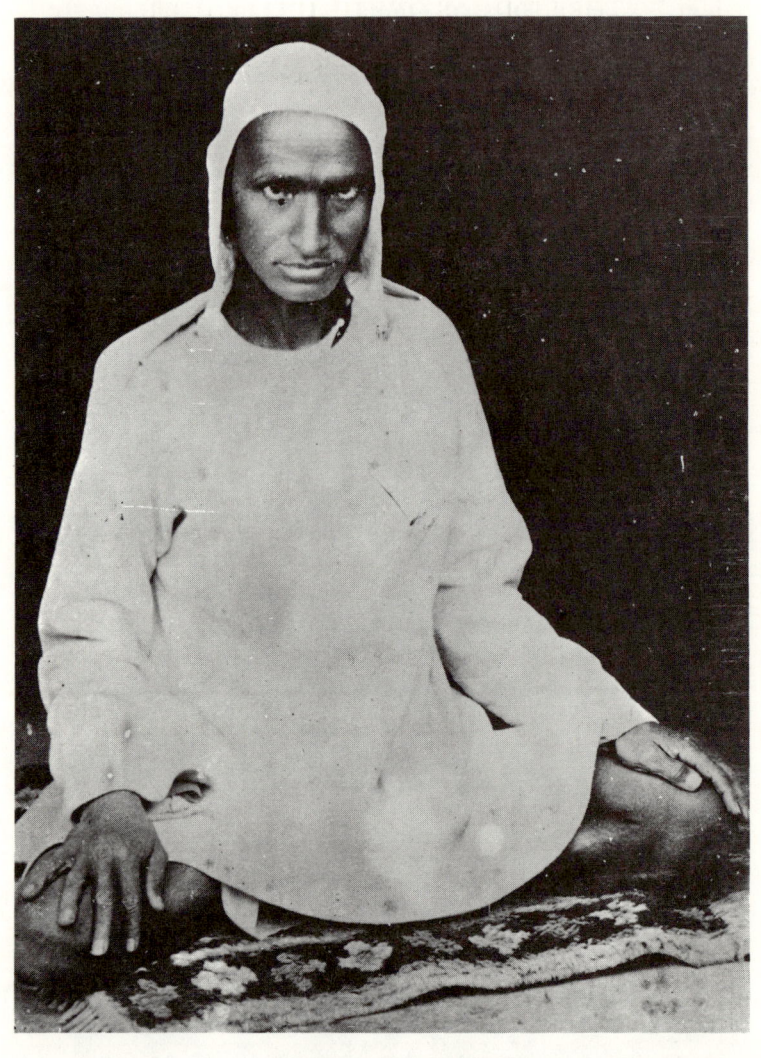

Sri Kairakhan Baba

THE SIDDHAS OF THE HIMALAYAS

The Himalayan region is considered to be a holy region and is associated with the names of deities, saints and great sages. It has been the home of the *Siddhas* for thousands of years and is said to possess a peculiar psychic atmosphere conducive to meditation and the practice of Yoga. Legends have it that the custodians of this planet's spiritual sciences have made this area their abode. From here they direct the regeneration of the world through telepathic influence, training special disciples who are then sent to work with people in society. All scriptures of India, which find their roots in the *Vedas*, refer to the Himalayas.

Paramahansa Yogananda, in his *Autobiography of a Yogi*, first told the world of a great immortal known as Sri Babaji, who revealed himself to Lahiri Mahasaya in the sixth decade of the last century. The meeting took place near Ranikhet, an area long sanctified by saints and illumined masters. The authority of age lends a spiritual aura to various pilgrimage places in this area, and it is a place where many go to find peace and inner solace.

Because this area is ideal for quiet meditation, many saints, some who are known to the public and some who are not known, have visited here and performed what are considered to be miracles. Such demonstrations are not meant for publicity or personal gain, but they are sometimes useful in calling forth faith in sincere devotees of God. There are persons still living today who recall having personally witnessed the divine wonders of these saints, and it is an inspiration to listen to their stories.

One such saint is known to more recent devotees as Sri Hairakhan Baba, and many consider this saint to be the same person as Babaji, who initiated Lahiri Mahasaya. The stories told are similar, and thousands of persons in India take for granted that this *avatara* has appeared in different places at different times and been known by various names. As Hairakhan Baba, he arrived in the small village of Hairakhan, in Naini Tal district, and there settled in 1894. No one knew who he was or from whence he had journied. Thus, the people called him Hairakhan Baba, "the revered father of Hairakhan." The village had been so named, because a great many myrobalan (*harra*) grew there. Myrobalan fruit is astringent and has several practical uses. Because of his style of dress at that time and the fact that he spoke a dialect which was a mixture of *Kumaonee Pahari* and *Nepali Doti*, he was considered to have come from Nepal. A manuscript written by him contains what appear to be a mixture of Pali and Tibetan characters. His age was unknown, though there were the remains of scars on his body, and he was assumed to have been in his body since the great *Mahabharata* wars.

Sri Hairakhan Baba was obviously an accomplished master of *Yoga*, since he was observed to remain rapt in immense peace and calm—a permanent experience of *samadhi*. For about thirty-five years, this saint remained in the area, visiting villages, towns and roaming about the countryside. Wherever he went, people flocked to him for *darshan*, his divine blessing. He was considered by them as a perfect Incarnation of the Supreme. Sri Hairakhan Baba practiced strict disciplines and possessed great yogic powers, which he used to bring good fortune to people and to heal many of their ailments. He is known to have restored sight to the blind and to have raised up persons near death. He could control the elements and was said to "ride the air," as he could cover great distances in a short period of time. He was known to appear in the flesh in more than two places at the same time, and he could use water, instead of clarified butter (*ghee*), to pour into ceremonial fires. When he did this, he said that he "looked for the *ghee* in the water." Since everything has subtle elements in combination, he could call forth the mixture of available subtle elements from any substance and use it according to his will. When Lahiri Mahasaya was with Babaji decades before, he reported that those close to Babaji often did not need to prepare their meals, since the master would point to a container and whatever food a disciple wanted would instantly appear therein.

The most intricate questions dealing with religion and philosophy were easily answered by Sri Hairakhan Baba. His teachings were universal and applicable to persons of all religions. Public rituals and ceremonies were encouraged for the welfare of the people and to encourage a harmonious working relationship with the forces of nature and the intelligent beings on subtle planes. *Siddhas* know *mantras* and prayer formulas which enable them to use sound frequency to contact the higher realms and to bring those energies into this physical realm. Frequently, when asked by a person if one's personal problem would be solved, the saint would say: "Your wish will be fulfilled if you sincerely rely upon God or the Highest Reality."

Before leaving the area, Sri Hairakhan Baba toured a number of Himalayan areas, concluding his travels at the border town of Askote. He then bade farewell to those who had accompanied him and crossed over the river to Nepal. He did not return in his physical form, although reports of his activities in Nepal were received by disciples. While in the Himalayas, he established several *Siddha* ashrams which are used to this day. Some are located at Katgharia, Shitlakhet (near Almora) and Naini Tal.

Babaji is still considered to move about the area in his subtle form, keeping his promise to remain on earth for the duration of this present cycle. In 1950 a saint known as Mahendra Brahmachari came to this area and visited several of the ashrams founded by the great *avatara*. While meditating at these places, he had visions of Babaji in his light form. In 1952 Mahendra Brahmachari again visited Babaji's ashram at Sai Debi, near Ranikhet, and saw the divine light form in daylight. In 1958 temples were built at Katgharia and at Brindaban and consecrated to Babaji. On both occasions, during the consecration ceremonies, thousands of persons saw a mass of light moving about the open spaces near the temples. The light, about four feet high and two feet wide, hovered over the ground as it moved.

In 1942, a Swedish artist and philosopher, Neils O'Lief Chresendor decided to visit Almora district in India. He had once had a vision of Babaji while visiting Moscow in Russia. His statue of Babaji is now enshrined in a temple in Kausani.

A contemparary of Sri Hairakhan Baba was the saint known as Sombari Baba. Every Monday (*Sombar*) this holy man would welcome people to his ashram for his blessing and provide food for all. Sometimes the number of those gathered would be one thousand, and there was always enough food for everyone. Sombari Baba himself ate only one or two small flour cakes which were baked over a fire. Scraps of left-over food were distributed to the animals, birds and fish nearby.

Wearing only a loin cloth and a light blanket, Sombari Baba practiced extreme yogic disciplines and was a master of *pranayama*. His main ashram was in Padampuri, and another was located in Kakarighat, by the side of a river. He, too, could control the elements and cause small quantities of food to be extended to meet whatever need was presented. He would place holy ash from a nearby fire on the forehead of devotees as they took leave to return to their homes. Sombari Baba held Sri Hairakhan Baba in high regard and often said that the gods and goddesses in subtle realms bowed down at the mention of his name. Hairakhan, likewise, spoke highly of Sombari Baba and praised his yogic attainment.

When Sombari Baba prepared to depart his physical form, he called one of his closest devotees to the ashram and informed the devotee of his plan. He gave instructions for his body to be cremated with correct rites. The

Masters of Yoga

next day the saint's body was found, an aura of serenity pervading the space around it.

Also, prior to his own *mahasamadhi*, Sombari Baba told of another *Siddha* who would come to this region. About two years later, in 1921, a young saint was found to be residing in a nearby cave, and he became known as Bal Brahmachari Maharaj. The saint was youthful, appeared to be in his late teens, had long golden hair and bright, shining eyes. Especially after his daily practice of *Yoga* and *pranayama*, his whole body would glow. He could chant the verses in Sanskrit from any of the great epics, the *Vedas* and the *Shastras*. His vast knowledge, almost impossible to believe for one so youthful, enabled him to perform ritual ceremonies with correct and precise scriptural rites and *mantras*. Devotees of the area accepted Bal Brahmachari Maharaj as being in the spirit and tradition of Sri Sombari Baba, because of the similarity of yogic power expressed and because Sombari Baba had foretold of him.

As with the case of so many *Siddhas* who came to this area, the young saint's background was not known. He generally conversed in Hindi but sometimes spoke in the Kumaoni dialect mixed with Nepali words. Bal Brahmachari usually taught in a subtle manner, giving hints for listeners to perceive and to apply in their lives. He could also heal through yogic knowledge and, in many ways, quietly blessed the people of the area with his presence. He usually lived simply and was disciplined in his daily practices. When he traveled to distant places and moved among the public, he wore ordinary clothes so as not to stand out as a holy man.

The saint stayed at various ashrams and sactified them with his presence, including the ashrams used earlier by both Sombari Baba and Hairakhan Baba. In 1959, through yogic *pranayama* (a method used to draw the currents of the body upward at the time of transition) Bal Brahmachari entered *mahasamadhi*. There are no known photographs of him.

It is of interest to note that frequently, when a new

young *Siddha* appears only a few years after the departure of one who is considered truly divine, the new one is believed to be the former one who has returned in a new body, and is accepted as such. We are told that some *Siddhas* "remain in the body" for centuries, moving from place to place as the need is revealed. They renew the body through the practice of advanced *kriyas*. Sometimes they appear to age and then either depart the area or leave the body, only to return in a few years in a new vital form. Whether such a soul actually retains the physical form and rejuvenates it or leaves the form and returns in a new one is of little consequence. Such *Siddhas*, who have a responsibility to remain in contact with planet earth, always remain in their subtle form, so the matter of how they handle the body (retaining it or discarding it for a new one) is merely a matter of personal decision. Satya Sai Baba, for instance, left the physical form known as Shirdi Sai Baba and has said that he will leave his present form when it becomes ninety-five years of age, in order to return in a new form which will be known as Prema Sai Baba. As a fully conscious being, he can do this with clear intention. Sometimes, between physical form appearances, *Siddhas* rest in *samadhi* or work on inner planes for a while. Yoganandaji told us he would return in a new body and spend some time with Babaji in the Himalayas. He also told us that some of us would be with him there at a later time, after our outward mission is fulfilled. Lamas of Tibet are also known to have the ability to plan future incarnations, and there has been a close working relationship between the Himalayan *Siddhas* and several of the Lamas.

My *guru* told of many *Siddhas* whose work goes unnoticed to the outer world but who, nevertheless, play an important role in the evolutionary process. I have mentioned here only a few of them and, doubtless, in the future more information will be shared, when the time is right for it to be known. What little is made known is for the purpose of inspiring true seekers and for giving assurance to those who occasionally wonder about the future of the planet and of mankind's place in the cosmic scheme. Regardless of the culture in which a *Siddha* master works, his emphasis is the same. He comes to remind us all of God and of the innate potential we all have to know Him.

Om Bhagavan Gurudev Ji!

GLOSSARY

The following one hundred Sanskrit words are ones which are commonly used in Yoga books and philosophical texts. An understanding of their meanings will help the student to derive greater insight into various works studied. Other Sanskrit words and terms will be found explained in the text matter of this book.

Advaita—Non-duality: the teaching that God, soul and the universe are One. Known as *Vedanta*; the final summation of the *Vedas*.

ahamkara—The ego, or "I" consciousness.

ajna—The "plexus of command" or third eye center.

ajnana—Meaning either individual or cosmic ignorance. This alone is said to be the cause of false perception and delusion.

akasa—Often spelled "Akasha"; the first of five material elements making up nature; sometimes translated as *ether*.

ananda—Bliss; often used as part of a monastic name of swamis. For instance, Yogananda: "bliss through Yoga or divine union."

anandamayakosa—The initial subtle sheath of the soul.

annamayakosa—The "food sheath" or physical body.

antahkarana—The inner organ of the soul's perception when operating in space and time; comprised of mind, intellect, ego-sense and feeling.

ashram—A secluded place for the practice of yogic disciplines or spiritual training.

Atman—A ray of Supreme Consciousness shining in the organ of the intellect of the mind. A particularization of Supreme Consciousness.

avadhuta—A supremely Self-Realized soul who functions through a mind and body but whose consciousness extends to the Infinite.

avatara—The "descent" of Divinity into a human form; a Divine Incarnation; A Savior or World Redeemer.

avidya—Meaning "Not knowledge"; lack of understanding of the nature of Consciousness and Its manifestations.

Ayurveda—Scripture of Life; an ancient Indian science of medicine and health principles.

Bhagavan—Lord; literally one endowed with the six attributes: infinite spiritual power, righteousness, glory, splendor, knowledge and renunciation. Used in reference to a fully Self-Realized person.

Bhagavad-Gita—An eighteen chapter work: "The Song of God." One of the central yogic scriptures setting forth the conversation between Krishna (an Incarnation of God) and Arjuna (the seeker on the path of Yoga).

Bhakti—Devotion; intense love for God.

Brahma—The first person in the Trinity in Hindu thought; the same as "God the Father" of the Christian tradition.

Brahmachari—A self-disciplined student who devotes himself to spiritual practices under a guru.

Brahmaloka—The abode of God; corresponding to the highest plane of heaven this side of the Transcendental Field.

Brahman—The Supreme Reality; the Absolute, without attributes or characteristics.

Brahma-Sutras—Also known as the *Vedanta-Sutras*; a treatise on high philosophical views and a central scripture for students whose quest is the path of knowledge.

Glossary

Brahmavidya—The knowledge of Supreme Consciousness.

buddhi—The faculty of discernment or determination; sometimes defined as "intellect," that which makes decisions.

chakra—A subtle center for psychic energy in the central pathway of the spinal cord; also the distribution center through which energies flow. The word means "wheel."

Chiti—The Absolute in Its creative and dynamic aspect as power.

chitta—The individual consciousness which perceives differences in Universal Being; it mediates between the inner and the outer realms.

deva—A "god" or shining one. Gods and goddesses (*devis*) dwell in subtle realms.

dhyana—Flowing the attention to one point during meditation; the sixth stage in Raja Yoga practice. Next comes *dharana*, pure meditation, followed by *samadhi* or the peak experience.

diksha—Yogic initiation, during which time instruction is given in a precise meditation method and the guru transmits his *shakti* into the disciple.

Govinda—One of the names for Krishna.

guna—The qualities or electric attributes in nature. *Tamas guna* stands for inertia or heaviness; *rajas guna* is the neutralizing current, sometimes referred to as the active quality; *sattva guna* promotes righteousness and spiritual enlightenment.

Guru—Literally "darkness" and "light"; that which dispells the darkness from the mind and consciousness of the seeker. The *Guru* is considered as God in human form Who comes for the welfare of the disciple on the path.

Gurukripa—The grace of God flowing through the *Guru*.

Guruseva—Service to the *Guru* is considered service to God. Through attunement with the *Guru* one identifies with his consciousness and experiences liberation.

ida—Left *nadi* or channel through which vital current flows; the moon current or negative polarity.

Isvara—Or "Iswara," the personal aspect of God which governs and controls the universe. Supreme Consciousness *as* the ruler of the manifest worlds.

japa—Repetition of any of the names of God for the purpose of meditation and concentration.

Jivanmukta—A free soul; one who is liberated while yet working through the body. Remaining *karma* may still persist but the person is inwardly free.

jnana—Jnana Yoga is the way to freedom through discernment. The word means "knowledge" of that contemplated.

jnani—One who is possessed of highest knowledge.

karma—Action; sometimes translated as "duty"; for instance, "It is my *karma* to do this work." Also, used in the explanation of cause and effect in the phenomenal universe.

Khechari Mudra—The state in which one is free to roam in the spaces in consciousness; also the physical act where the tongue is drawn up into the nasal pharynx, stimulating a discharge of fluids from the cranial region.

Kriya Yoga—Yogic kriyas are spontaneous purification actions on subtle levels which take place when *kundalini* is awakened. *Kriya Yoga* also refers to the precise system of meditation techniques taught by my line of gurus as advised by Mahavatar Babaji.

kundalini—Dormant, static, vital force resting in nature; when it awakens in nature, then life emerges on the planet. When it awakens in man, then the soul be-

Glossary 187

gins its journey through inner space in the direction of Self-Realization.

Maha—Literally means "great," such as in *Mahatma* or "great soul."

Mahadeva—"Great god," often used in reference to *Shiva*.

mahasamadhi—The final conscious departure of a *yogi* from his physical form. Also, used in reference to the shrine which is erected over the body after transition.

manas—The aspect of the mind which is the seat or root of the five senses. When the soul identifies with *manas*, it is described as "man."

manomayakosa—The sheath or covering of the mind.

mantra—Sound used for its specific influence on its environment: physical, mental or more subtle. Can be intoned audibly, mentally recited or listened to in deep meditation.

maya—Sometimes referred to as the "stuff" of which the worlds are formed; the cause of illusion. Made up of time, space, light particles and the primal energy of OM. *Maya* has two characteristics: it forms as the world, and it veils truth from the soul.

moksha—Liberation or freedom from *maya*.

mudra—A symbolic pose or gesture; a "seal"; a yogic practice used to awaken *kundalini* and to gain control over vital processes.

nada—Different inner sounds heard during meditation which are variations of the primal sound of OM. *Nadayoga* is the science of sound.

nadi—A channel through which prana flows in the psychic system.

nadi-shuddhi—Purification of the nerves and subtle channels due to the active flowing of *shakti* after *kundalini* is awakened.

Nirguna Brahman—Supreme Consciousness without attributes or qualities.

Nirvana—To "blow out" or to eradicate from the mind all that prevents the clear perception of Reality. To attain *nirvana* is to be liberated as a result of all subtle impressions of the mind having been erased.

Nirvikalpa Samadhi—The experience of Pure Consciousness without mental or conceptual support. This *samadhi* is not pure or permanent, according to some, unless all latent impressions of the mind are removed.

OM—The primal sound from which all outer appearances manifest. The *Pranava, Aum* or *Amen*.

Paramahansa—The highest title for a Self-Realized *yogi*. One who rests in God-Realization and is not touched by the world process.

pingala—Right spinal pathway for flowing *prana*. The "sun" current, as opposed to the "moon" current of *ida*. The positive flow of current in the system. When both currents are neutralized, then *kundalini* can ascend.

Prakriti—The material realms (nature) consisting of the elements and electric attributes or qualities.

prana—Vital force animating the universe and all forms. All *pranas* are divisions of the Sound Current.

pranayama—Regulation of vital forces, usually through conscious regulation of breathing and specific *mudras*.

pranamayakosa—The vital body or astral sheath of the soul.

prarabdha karma—Subconscious impressions now beginning to manifest or to be worked out in this incarnation.

Purusha—Conscious Principle, which unites with subtle elements in nature to form the material realms.

Glossary

rajas—The principle of activity or neutralization.

rasa-lila—The eternal "dance" taking place between the Lord of the universe and individual souls.

rishi—A seer; one who reveals the wisdom of the scriptures.

sadhana—Spiritual disciplines of *Yoga*.

Saguna Brahman—Supreme Consciousness with attributes; the Godhead, with three aspects: Existence, Intelligence and Creative Energy.

sahasrara—The center of consciousness in the cerebrum; the highest of the seven *chakras* and the one which is superior to them all.

samadhi—When the waves of the mind cease and "oneness" is experienced. Lower *samadhi* is oneness with an object (saguna); higher *samadhi* is without any object (nirguna).

samasara—The "forever becomingness" of the world process. One who is deluded and identified with change is sure to suffer from unwanted change of circumstances and relationships. To identify with the world process is to be bound to the "wheel of rebirth" and to rise above identification is to be free.

Sanatana Dharma—The Eternal Religion or the eternal way of righteousness. Can be traced to pre-*Vedic* times and is said to be without origin, having always been known to a few initiates.

sannyasin—A renunciate who has taken holy vows (*sannyasa*) for the purpose of devoting all energies to Self-Realization and world service.

sattva—The elevating attribute of nature, that which leads one to *Sat*, the pure truth.

Shakti—The cosmic energy which forms the worlds and maintains them; the energy awakened in one who receives *kundalini* initiation.

Shaktipat—The infusion of energy from *guru* to disciple which can take place during initiation or spontaneously when the disciple is receptive to the experience.

Shambhavi mudra—When the attention is focused spontaneously and one's attention is flowing to the Divine nature, whether the eyes are open or closed. When the attention does not flutter.

Shiva—Third person in the Hindu Trinity; the aspect of the Godhead which sends forth Creative Energy and then dissolves It. *Shiva* is the patron diety of *Yoga*.

Siddha—A "perfect being" who is accomplished in *Yoga*. A true Master who can awaken *shakti* and lead the disciple to liberation of consciousness.

siddhis—Powers of perfection as a result of soul awakening.

sushumna—Central pathway through which *kundalini* ascends to the crown *chakra*, resulting in evolutionary transformation of the system and the highest *samadhi*.

tattva—The true or inner essence of a thing. The essence of the senses are the roots of the senses on the subtle level. The essence of the worlds is God, the Light behind the "darkness' of outer manifestation. The essence of a thing is known only when one turns the attention to the source of the appearance.

Turiya—The "fourth" state of consciousness; transcending the three states of waking, dream and deep sleep.

Upanishads—A section of the *Vedas*, which are considered an important collection of scripture. These scriptures were taught in the oral tradition, by word of mouth, for hundreds of years before being written in Sanskrit.

Vedanta—The summing up of the wisdom of the *Vedas*. The usual declaration regarding the nature of a person or any appearance is: *Tat Twam Asi*—"That

Glossary

Thou Art!" Supreme Consciousness is the cause and support of all that appears.

Vishnu—The second person in the Trinity. The aspect of the Godhead which maintains order and preserves the universe.

viveka—Discrimination between the changeless and the transitory.

Vyasa—A sage who is believed to have arranged the *Vedas* in their present form. Legend has it that the name refers to several sages who worked on the project over a period of time.

Yoga—To "yoke" or join together. The complete system of various compatible disciplines which enable one to harmonize conflicting and active currents in the system so that the light of the soul can be directly cognized.

Center for Spiritual Awareness has world headquarters in northeast Georgia. Here on a ten-acre site are found the spacious education building, administrative offices, residence homes, library and meditation temple. CSA is not a commune, nor is it a spiritual community in the usually accepted sense. It is a service center from which literature and training aids flow to a waiting world, and a retreat center to which seekers come for instruction and spiritual refreshment.

If you would like informative literature about books, recordings and available programs, you have but to contact the CSA office. There is no obligation. We are here to serve you as you unfold your inborn divine potential. Contact: Center for Spiritual Awareness, Lake Rabun Road, Post Office Box 7, Lakemont, Georgia 30552.